Spanish

FOR THE PHARMACY PROFESSIONAL

Notices

The authors and publisher have made every effort to ensure the accuracy and completeness of the information presented in this book. However, the authors and publisher cannot be held responsible for the continued currency of the information, any inadvertent errors or omissions, or the application of this information. Therefore, the authors and publisher shall have no liability to any person or entity with regard to claims, loss, or damage caused or alleged to be caused, directly or indirectly, by the use of information contained herein.

The inclusion in this book of any product in respect to which patent or trademark rights may exist shall not be deemed, and is not intended as, a grant of or authority to exercise any right or privilege protected by such patent or trademark. All such rights or trademarks are vested in the patent or trademark owner, and no other person may exercise the same without express permission, authority, or license secured from such patent or trademark owner.

The inclusion of a brand name does not mean the authors or the publisher has any particular knowledge that the brand listed has properties different from other brands of the same product, nor should its inclusion be interpreted as an endorsement by the authors or the publisher. Similarly, the fact that a particular brand has not been included does not indicate the product has been judged to be in any way unsatisfactory or unacceptable. Further, no official support or endorsement of this book by any federal or state agency or pharmaceutical company is intended or inferred.

Readers

To listen to the audio components of this book, go to www.pharmacist.com/SPANISH.

Instructors

To obtain the Instructor's Guide for this book, e-mail your request to the publisher at aphabooks@aphanet.org.

Spanish

FOR THE PHARMACY PROFESSIONAL

Jeri J. Sias, PharmD
Clinical Associate Professor
UTEP/UT Austin Cooperative Pharmacy Program
University of Texas at El Paso
El Paso, Texas

Susana V. James, MFA
Independent Instructor and Translator
El Paso, Texas

Cristina Cabello C. de Martínez, PhD
Senior Lecturer
Department of Spanish and Portuguese
University of Texas at Austin
Austin, Texas

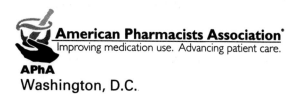
American Pharmacists Association®
Improving medication use. Advancing patient care.
APhA
Washington, D.C.

Acquiring Editor: Sandra J. Cannon
Managing Editor: Ashley Young, Publications Professionals LLC
Copy Editors: Laura Glassman and Linda Stringer, Publications Professionals LLC
Proofreader: Jennifer Thompson, Publications Professionals LLC
Book Design and Layout: Circle Graphics
Cover Design: Richard Muringer, APhA Creative Services

©2009 by the American Pharmacists Association
Published by the American Pharmacists Association
1100 15th Street, NW, Suite 400
Washington, DC 20005-1707
www.pharmacist.com

APhA was founded in 1852 as the American Pharmaceutical Association

To comment on this book via e-mail, send your message to the publisher at aphabooks@aphanet.org

Library of Congress Cataloging-in-Publication Data

Sias, Jeri J.
  Spanish for the pharmacy professional / Jeri J. Sias, Susana V. James, Cristina Cabello C. de Martinez.
    p. ; cm.
  Includes bibliographical references.
  Text in English and Spanish.
  ISBN 978-1-58212-120-8
  1. Spanish language—Conversation and phrase books (for medical personnel) 2. Pharmacy—Terminology.
I. James, Susana V. II. Martinez, Cristina Cabello C. de. III. American Pharmacists Association. IV. Title.
  [DNLM: 1. Pharmaceutical Preparations—Phrases—English. 2. Pharmaceutical Preparations—Phrases—Spanish.
3. Patient Education as Topic—Phrases—English. 4. Patient Education as Topic—Phrases—Spanish. 5. Pharmaceutical
Services—Phrases—English. 6. Pharmaceutical Services—Phrases—Spanish. 7. Pharmacy—methods—Phrases—English.
8. Pharmacy—methods—Phrases—Spanish. QV 15 S562s 2009]

PC4120.M3S53 2009
468.3'42102461—dc22

Printed in Canada   2008047738

Índice
Contents

Prefacio
Preface

Approximately 12% of the U.S. population 5 years of age or older speaks Spanish in the home, with some areas of the country at a much higher percentage.[1] With these changes in language demographics in the United States, the pharmacy community has an opportunity to respond by learning to communicate basic medication information to patients in Spanish. This textbook, *Spanish for the Pharmacy Professional*, has been developed, used in the classroom, and revised since 2001. Students using this text have ranged from non-Spanish speakers to native Spanish-language speakers. In the process of creating this text, the authors have focused on balancing the use of culturally appropriate Spanish (with a focus on Mexican Spanish) with technical Spanish that is practical for the pharmacist.

The original course and text were developed alongside pharmacy courses for nonprescription products and pharmacy patient assessment. The primary intent was to provide students with examples in Spanish on how to counsel patients on various medication formulations and to perform basic assessment common to pharmacy practice. To develop the initial dialogues, the American Pharmacists Association's *Handbook of Nonprescription Drugs* and the Prime Questions (developed through the Indian Health Service) were used as guides.[2,3] These materials were supplemented with prescription product information and other material to cover various formulations and assessment techniques.

Patient–pharmacist relationship and the Hispanic culture

For many patients in the Hispanic culture, it is important to recognize the values of respect and family, the personal relationship between patients and health care personnel, and the importance of nonverbal communication.[4] When one is counseling patients, being respectful and providing basic expressions of courtesy can be key to establishing and developing the patient–pharmacist relationship. Many Spanish-speaking patients will appreciate the effort of, and even expect, pharmacy personnel to take time for small talk before providing medication information. Attempts to make introductions, to say "Hello" and "How are you and your family" in Spanish, and even to shake hands or make a gesture toward the patient can help to create a rapport. Once a rapport is established, the patient (and the patient's family) may feel more comfortable continuing to trust in the professional relationship. Some basic expressions of courtesy are provided in the text and dialogues.

Goals

The primary goal of this text is to provide tools for pharmacy personnel to communicate basic medication information to Spanish speakers while confirming patient understanding (Prime Questions from the Indian Health Service). The text and dialogues have been designed to

- Include basic pharmacy vocabulary.
- Explain steps to counsel on a variety of medication formulations (e.g., patches, suppositories).
- Provide general questions for common self-care problems and disease states.
- Provide some key phrases and vocabulary for physical assessment that are more commonly used by pharmacists (e.g., blood pressure).
- Provide cultural notes relevant to various segments of the Hispanic community.

About the text

The text is based in standard Spanish. It is highly influenced by the Mexican culture because it was created on the U.S.-Mexico border. Spanish-speaking cultures have many other dialects, expressions, and vocabulary from other areas (e.g., Cuba, Puerto Rico, Central and South America, and Spain), and so regional variations will exist. The authors welcome feedback for including expressions and cultural notes from other Spanish-speaking cultures.

This text is not a grammar book, but it does include some grammar exercises and short explanations to promote better understanding of the structure of the Spanish language. Grammar cannot be ignored in learning Spanish. However, when one is learning and speaking technical Spanish, perfect grammar is not expected.

The patient-counseling phrases incorporate the use of the formal "you" (*usted*) in Spanish and use the verb conjugation form of commands (*mandatos*). These forms are the most respectful way of speaking to an adult patient. The verbs in each chapter are conjugated in the "I" (*yo*), the formal "you" (*usted*), and the command (imperative) form (*mandato*). These are the most common ways that a pharmacist will likely conjugate verbs to communicate with an adult patient.

Because grammar explanations are not covered thoroughly, the authors advise that a grammar book and verb conjugation book be used as a reference. Pronunciation has not been provided; however, audio of most of the book's vocabulary and dialogues is available on the publisher's Web site at www.pharmacist.com/SPANISH. In some sections, the Spanish may appear to be written at an advanced level. The authors worked to start with a more basic Spanish and to build in difficulty throughout the text. The questions and counseling points given by pharmacy personnel are written at a more basic level. Because patients will not talk

only in the present tense, the audio dialogues are written in a more natural, conversational style.

Textbook structure

The textbook is divided into four primary sections: introductory vocabulary, chapters on medication use, physical assessment, and appendixes and grammar. The introduction includes pharmacy terminology, medication formulations, and units of measurement, as well as dialogues on greeting patients, gathering patient health and medication information, and answering the telephone. The first four chapters focus on diverse oral formulations of medications, such as tablets, syrups, and powders. The final six chapters focus on non-oral or different formulations, including eye and ear products, topical formulations, vaginal and rectal products, patches, inhalers, and subcutaneous injections.

Each chapter includes verb vocabulary (conjugated in common forms that are practical for pharmacists), other vocabulary, questions and counseling points in the form of dialogues, cultural notes, and some practice exercises. Cultural notes were created on the basis of experiences of the authors and published literature.

There are two forms of the dialogues in each lesson and chapter. The first dialogue is more straightforward and includes the new vocabulary for the chapter. Students are encouraged to work with their class instructor to adapt the counseling questions and to use vocabulary appropriate to their language level and the needs of their community. The second dialogue is an audio dialogue transcript and follows the general outline in the first dialogue while providing a more comprehensive counseling session. Verb tenses and vocabulary outside of the chapter vocabulary are used in the audio dialogues to simulate how patients might respond to a pharmacist.

Some lessons are grouped into chapters around similar health problems or disease states and include introductory questions about the condition. To help limit the length of the lessons, other chapters that include more information about medication use (e.g., inhalers, suppositories) do not include introductory questions. Once vocabulary is introduced in a lesson or chapter, it is generally not repeated in a subsequent chapter.

Vocabulary and short phrases related to physical assessment common in pharmacy practice are provided. The appendixes provide some brief information on days of the week, numbers, and common questions. The grammar notes include a brief section focusing on the commonly used verb tenses and conjugations found in the text. A glossary of most of the vocabulary found in the text is also included. An instructor's guide accompanies the text and includes a course guide, written exam and answer bank, pharmacy-based listening exercises, and oral exam samples.

Note to instructors

The authors recommend that the text be taught by a Spanish-language instructor with the assistance of a faculty member who is a pharmacist (consult Instructor's Guide). The instructor should have full command of the Spanish language in order to teach technical terms in a professional dialogue, to understand the subtle cultural notes necessary for the pharmacy setting, and to address grammar questions that arise. Spanish-language instructors with technical language experience in the medical field would be ideal. The pharmacist instructor will be able to provide practical information to the classroom or workshop setting about medication information. The pharmacist is encouraged to provide sample medications and formulations to the class so that students can have hands-on practice. Furthermore, the pharmacist can update information about products and assist with preparation of counseling props if needed.

Although the authors have taught the course with beginners, they highly recommend that, if possible, students have at least 1 year of college-level Spanish or that pharmacy professionals have taken a community course in basic Spanish conversation and grammar. It is the authors' experience that the first month of class is often very difficult for students new to the Spanish language and requires extensive basic grammar supplementation. After one month, students gravitate to the process for counseling patients and using grammar in a functional way. Students should be reminded that their first pharmacy classes involved learning the "language of pharmacy" and that through study, repetition, and application, pharmacy material became more comprehensible. The process of learning a language also requires study, repetition, and application.

It is also critical for the instructor to provide feedback to the students regarding their Spanish-language limitations and skills for both speaking and writing before (through preassessment) and at the end of the course. The ideal pharmacy practice setting will provide access to a trained or certified Spanish-language interpreter (oral) and translator (written). This text does not provide information on how to use an interpreter.

Note to students

Many of the English translations of the Spanish dialogues are translated more literally to help the student understand the context and structure of the Spanish language. The authors have intentionally separated the Spanish dialogues from their English translations. If students review only the Spanish dialogue or if the English translation is readily available, students may just read the dialogue. However, if students review the English translation separately from the Spanish, they are forced to think of how they would functionally communicate with patients.

Students should remember that interacting with patients involves two-way communication. It is possible for the student to give information and never know if the patient understands. Therefore, being able to have the patient repeat information and demonstrate use of medication is important.

The text includes exercises for reading, listening, and writing. However, the student must practice speaking and using the language in context as much as possible! Also, students are encouraged to look up vocabulary and phrases in other Spanish-language sources to enhance their learning. As students progress, they should also realize their own limitations in the Spanish language so as to avoid errors. Using a fully bilingual Spanish-English interpreter is appropriate and recommended. Many Spanish-only speakers will still appreciate the efforts of the pharmacy team to communicate greetings and basic information in Spanish even if an interpreter is used.

It is impossible to cover every patient-counseling situation. However, by the end of this course, pharmacy students and personnel should have developed a strong enough understanding of the language to be able to adapt to most pharmacy medication counseling situations. The authors encourage instructors to give students homework to practice other medication counseling and pharmacy work situations.

Conclusion

Using a second language in the professional setting is challenging; however, the authors believe that dedicated students of this text will, at the very minimum, be able to provide in Spanish basic expressions of courtesy and clarify for patients the appropriate understanding and use of most medication formulations while enjoying some of the subtleties of the Spanish language and of Hispanic cultures. *¡Mucho éxito!*

REFERENCES
1. U.S. Census Bureau data. Available at: http://factfinder.census.gov/.
2. Berardi RR, DeSimone EM, Newton GD, et al., eds. *Handbook of Nonprescription Drugs*. 13th ed. Washington, DC: American Pharmaceutical Association; 2002.
3. Gardner M, Boyce RW, Herrier RN. *Pharmacist–Patient Consultation Program PPCP-Unit I: An Interactive Approach to Verifying Patient Understanding*. New York: Pfizer Educational Services; 1991.
4. National Alliance for Hispanic Health. *Delivering Health Care to Hispanics: A Manual for Providers*. 4th ed. Washington, DC: Estrella Press; 2007.

Acknowledgments

To our families (*a nuestras familias*)

To the patients and community members living in El Paso, Texas, who unknowingly helped shape and guide the approach to developing this textbook

To Louis "Cliff" Littlefield, Magdalena Red, Lisa Meyer, Stephanie Valdez, José O. Rivera, Gloria Pinto, Joanne Richards, and Patrick Davis for their assistance and support in developing the first drafts of this text

To the faculty, staff, and students of the University of Texas at El Paso/University of Texas at Austin Cooperative Pharmacy Program and University of Texas at Austin College of Pharmacy who have assisted in reviewing parts of the text and taking the first versions of the course

To the Health Resources Services Administration–Hispanic Center of Excellence at the University of Texas at Austin College of Pharmacy for initial funding to support the expansion and revision of the course

To the University of Texas at Austin College of Pharmacy for the opportunity to create this curriculum

To the University of Texas at El Paso College of Health Sciences and the University of Texas Pan American for their commitment to serving the people in their communities

To La Fe Production Studio at Centro de Salud Familiar La Fe Inc. of El Paso, Texas, for providing the audio recording

Photography: Enrique J. James and Jeri J. Sias

Audio engineering: Marcos Hernández Jr.

Voice recording: Ana Laura Gamboa, Amando Enrique González-Stuart, Susana V. James, José O. Rivera, and Jeri J. Sias

Contributors

Jeri Sias, PharmD, is Clinical Associate Professor of Pharmacy with the University of Texas at El Paso/University of Texas at Austin Cooperative Pharmacy Program. Arriving in El Paso in 2000, she has used many of the methods found in the textbook to learn to function in the Spanish language. She uses Spanish in daily activities and counseling with patients in family practice settings. She provides the pharmacist expertise in catering the dialogues to clinical pharmacy experiences.

Susana James, MFA, is a Spanish-language instructor in the El Paso, Texas, area. She is from Mexico, has worked with medical personnel for many years, and has formerly owned a pharmacy in Mexico. She is knowledgeable in the common and formal language of medication. She has tutored and taught Spanish classes for pharmacy professionals since 1997.

Cristina Cabello de Martínez, PhD, is a Spanish-language instructor at the University of Texas at Austin and has taught medical Spanish to medical professionals and students for several years. She has taught the pharmacy course at the University of Texas at Austin since 2003, primarily to students of Spanish as a second language.

Introducción
Introduction

Presentación con el paciente / Meeting the patient

En la farmacia

FARMACÉUTICO(A): Buenos días. (Buenas tardes. Buenas noches.) Me llamo _____.
Soy el (la) farmacéutico(a). ¿Cómo se llama?

PACIENTE: *Me llamo _____.*

FARMACÉUTICO(A): Mucho gusto.

PACIENTE: *Igualmente.*

FARMACÉUTICO(A): ¿Cómo está? (¿Cómo ha estado?)

PACIENTE: *Más o menos bien, gracias.*

FARMACÉUTICO(A): ¿Cómo se siente?

PACIENTE: *Pues, mal.*

FARMACÉUTICO(A): ¿Cómo le puedo ayudar?

PACIENTE: *Fui con el doctor hoy y él me dio esta receta. Quiero comprar estas medicinas.*

FARMACÉUTICO(A): Sí, ahora mismo se las doy.

In the pharmacy*

PHARMACIST: Good morning. (Good afternoon. Good evening.) My name is _____. I am the pharmacist. What is your name?

PATIENT: *My name is _____.*

PHARMACIST: Pleased to meet you.

PATIENT: *Likewise.*

PHARMACIST: How are you? (How have you been?)

PATIENT: *More or less fine, thank you.*

PHARMACIST: How do you feel?

PATIENT: *Well, bad.*

PHARMACIST: How can I help you?

PATIENT: *I went to (with) the doctor today, and he gave me this prescription. I want to buy these medicines.*

PHARMACIST: Yes, I will give them to you right now.

---

*Not all the English translations throughout the book are written in standard English. Rather, they are a close literal translation from Spanish. This more literal translation can be a helpful teaching tool that allows the student to better understand grammatical rules and the arrangement of words (syntax) in the Spanish language.

▉ *Archivo electrónico del paciente / Computer patient information*

Fecha: _____

Sr./Sra./Srta.   Nombre: _____   Apellido: _____

Sexo: ☐ Femenino ☐ Masculino   Fecha de nacimiento: _____/_____/_____   Edad: _____
                                                         Mes/día/año

Dirección/domicilio: _____
Ciudad: _____ Estado: _____ Zona postal: _____

Teléfono (casa): _____ (celular): _____
Correo electrónico: _____ Ocupación/profesión: _____

Estado civil: ☐ Soltero(a)   ☐ Casado(a)   ☐ Divorciado(a)   ☐ Separado(a)   ☐ Viudo(a)

Nombre de su cónyuge o la persona que lo (la) cuida: _____
En caso de emergencia llamar a: _____
Relación: _____ Teléfono: _____

Número de seguro social: _____-____-_____ Compañía de seguro de salud: _____
Número de póliza (de medicamentos): _____

Reacción alérgica a medicamentos: _____

Fumador: ☐ Sí   ☐ No

Medicamentos:	Dosis	Frecuencia	Indicación
1._____	_____	_____	_____
2._____	_____	_____	_____
3._____	_____	_____	_____

Medicamentos sin receta: _____

Remedios naturales: _____

Inmunizaciones/vacunas (adulto): ☐ Gripe   ☐ Neumonía/pulmonía   ☐ Tétanos   Otra: _____
Fecha(s) recibida(s): _____

Historia familiar	Madre/padre	Historia familiar	Madre/padre
1._____	_____	2._____	_____

Médico(s): _____

Enfermedades crónicas	Fecha	Enfermedades crónicas	Fecha
1._____	_____	3._____	_____
2._____	_____	4._____	_____

Firma: _____ Fecha: _____

▨ *Archivo electrónico del paciente* / *Computer patient information*

Date: _____

Mr./Mrs./Miss   First name: _____   **Last name:** _____

Sex: ☐ Female ☐ Male   **Date of birth:** _____/_____/_____   **Age:** _____
                                              Month/day/year

Address: _____
City: _____   **State:** _____   **Zip code:** _____

Telephone (home): _____ **(cell):** _____
E-mail: _____ **Occupation/profession:** _____

Marital status: ☐ Single   ☐ Married   ☐ Divorced   ☐ Separated   ☐ Widowed

Name of spouse or caretaker: _____
Emergency contact number: _____
Relationship: _____ **Telephone:** _____

Social Security number: _____-_____-_____ **Health insurance carrier:** _____
Drug policy number: _____

Allergies to medications: _____

Smoker: ☐ Yes   ☐ No

Medications	Dosage	Frequency	Instructions
1._____	_____	_____	_____
2._____	_____	_____	_____
3._____	_____	_____	_____

Over-the-counter medications: _____

Herbal (natural) remedies: _____

Immunizations/vaccines (adult): ☐ Flu   ☐ Pneumonia   ☐ Tetanus   Other:_____
Date(s) received: _____

Family history	Mother/father	Family history	Mother/father
1._____	_____	2._____	_____

Doctor(s): _____

Chronic illnesses	Date	Chronic illnesses	Date
1._____	_____	3._____	_____
2._____	_____	4._____	_____

Signature: _____ **Date:** _____

Información del paciente / Patient information

	Spanish	English
1.	¿Qué fecha es hoy?	What is today's date?
2.	¿Cuál es su nombre? o ¿Cómo se llama?	What is your name?
3.	¿Cuál es su apellido paterno?	What is your last name (paternal)?
4.	¿Cuál es su fecha de nacimiento?	What is your date of birth?
5.	¿Qué edad tiene? o ¿Cuántos años tiene?	How old are you?
6.	¿Cuál es su dirección? o ¿Dónde vive?	What is your address? or Where do you live?
7.	¿En (De) qué ciudad? ¿En (De) qué estado?	In (From) what city? In (From) what state?
8.	¿Cuál es la zona postal de su domicilio?	What is your zip code?
9.	¿Cuál es su número de teléfono? ¿de celular? ¿su correo electrónico?	What is your telephone number? Your cell? Your e-mail address?
10.	¿Cuál es su ocupación (profesión)?	What is your occupation?
11.	¿Cuál es su estado civil?	What is your marital status?
12.	¿Cuál es el nombre de su cónyuge o la persona que lo (la) cuida?	What is the name of your spouse or caretaker?
13.	¿A quién podemos llamar en caso de emergencia?	Whom can we call in an emergency?
14.	¿Cuál es su relación con esta persona?	What is your relationship to this person?
15.	¿Cuál es el número de teléfono donde podemos localizar a esta persona?	What is the phone number where we can locate this person?
16.	¿Cuál es su número de seguro social?	What is your Social Security number?
17.	¿Cuál es el nombre de su compañía de seguro de salud?	What is your health insurance company?
18.	¿Cuál es su número de póliza (de medicamentos)?	What is your (medication) policy number?
19.	¿Tiene alergias a algún medicamento?	Do you have medication allergies?
20.	¿Es fumador(a)?	Are you a smoker?
21.	¿Actualmente qué medicamentos toma?	What medications do you currently take?
22.	¿Cuál es la dosis? ¿Con qué frecuencia los toma?	What is the dose? How often do you take them?
23.	¿Para qué los toma?	What are they for?
24.	¿Cuáles medicamentos sin receta toma?	What nonprescription medications do you take?
25.	¿Cuáles remedios naturales toma?	What herbal remedies do you take?
26.	¿Cuáles vacunas ha recibido como adulto? y ¿cuándo? ¿Contra la gripe? ¿la neumonía (pulmonía)? ¿Tétanos?	What vaccines have you received as an adult and when? Against influenza? Pneumonia? Tetanus?
27.	¿Qué tipo de enfermedades hay en su familia?	What types of diseases are there in your family?
28.	¿Por parte de su madre o de su padre?	On your mother's or your father's side?
29.	¿Quién es su médico?	Who is your doctor?
30.	¿Tiene enfermedades crónicas?	Do you have chronic diseases?
31.	¿Desde cuándo la(s) ha tenido?	How long have you had it (them)?
32.	Firme por favor al pie de la página (en la pantalla).	Sign at the bottom of the page (on the screen) please.

De la cultura / About the culture

1. In Spanish, a person legally uses two last names (paternal and maternal). The "first" last name is the paternal name and the one used for legal purposes in the United States. The "second" last name is the maternal name and recognizes the mother's family; it should not be used as the legal last name in the United States. Therefore, the correct way to address a patient who uses both last names on an application is to refer to him or her by the "first" last name.

   Example: José Manuel Rodríguez Juárez would be called Mr. Rodríguez.

2. In Latin America, the telephone number is often dictated in the following manner: 5-26-34-72 instead of 526-3472.

3. Many Hispanic patients are accustomed to saying and writing dates in a different form than is used in the United States. This difference can cause an error. For example, May 8, 2008, in Spanish is "8 de mayo del 2008." In the United States, the month is first followed by the day (e.g., 5/8/2008), but in Spanish-speaking countries, the day is first, then the month (e.g., 8/5/2008). It is important to clarify with the patient what is the month and what is the day, particularly when obtaining a date of birth.

Diálogo para el audio

PACIENTE: *Hola, buenos días. Mi nombre es Sonia Ramos. Vengo a recoger las medicinas de mi mamá, Lupita Salazar. ¿Están listas?*

TÉCNICO: Déjeme ver. Un momento por favor. ¿Cuándo trajo la receta?

PACIENTE: *Ella llamó ayer. Son sus medicamentos para la diabetes y para la presión.*

TÉCNICO: No, no pudimos surtirlas porque nos falta información. Necesito hacerle algunas preguntas.

PACIENTE: *Está bien.*

1. Hoy es 16 de septiembre del 2008.

2. ¿Cuál es el nombre completo de su mamá?
   Es Lupita Salazar Diego.

3. ¿Cuál es su apellido paterno?
   Es Salazar.

4. ¿Cuál es su fecha de nacimiento?
   El 6 de enero de 1942 (mil novecientos cuarenta y dos).

5. ¿Qué edad tiene?
   Tiene 66 (sesenta y seis) años.

6. ¿Cuál es su domicilio o dirección?
   Avenida López Anderson 1328 (trece veintiocho).

7. ¿De qué ciudad y estado?
   De aquí, de El Paso, Texas.

8. ¿Cuál es su zona postal?
   79902 (siete noventa y nueve–cero–dos).

9. ¿Cuál es su número de teléfono? ¿de celular? ¿su correo electrónico?
   6-11-24-69 (seis–once–veinticuatro–sesenta y nueve). No tiene celular, ni correo electrónico.

10. ¿Cuál es su ocupación o profesión?
    Ella es jubilada.

11. ¿Cuál es su estado civil?
    Es casada.

12. ¿Cuál es el nombre de su cónyuge o la persona que la cuida?
    Mi papá, Ignacio Diego.

    ¿Entonces su apellido es Salazar o Diego?
    Es Diego.

13. ¿A quién podemos llamar en caso de emergencia?
    A mí, Sonia Ramos.

14. Otra vez ¿cuál es su relación con la Señora Diego?
    Soy su hija.

15. ¿Cuál es su número de teléfono?
    2-56-28-39 (dos–cincuenta y seis–veintiocho–treinta y ocho).

16. ¿Cuál es el número de seguro social de su mamá?
    123-45-67-89 (ciento veintitrés–cuarenta y cinco–sesenta y siete–ochenta y nueve).

17. ¿Cuál es el nombre de su compañía de seguro de salud?
    Medicare.

18. ¿Cuál es su número de póliza (de medicamentos)?
    Es igual al del seguro social.

19. ¿Su mamá tiene alergias a algún medicamento?
    A la penicilina y a las sulfas.

20. ¿Es fumadora?
    No.

21. ¿Actualmente qué medicamentos toma?
    Creo que lisinopril y metformina.

22. ¿Cuál es la dosis? ¿Con qué frecuencia los toma?
    De 10 (diez) miligramos(mg) y de 500 (quinientos) mg. Toma sus medicamentos una vez al día.

23. ¿Para qué los toma?
    Para controlar su presión y la diabetes.

24. ¿Cuáles son los medicamentos sin receta que toma?
    Una aspirina de 81 mg.

25. ¿Cuáles son los remedios naturales que toma?
    Té de manzanilla.

26. ¿Cuáles son las vacunas que ha recibido como adulto? ¿Contra la gripe? ¿la neumonía (pulmonia)? ¿Tétanos?
    La llevé a otra farmacia para una vacuna contra la gripe en octubre.

27. ¿Tiene algunos riesgos de enfermedades en su familia?
    Pues hay mucha gente que tiene diabetes en nuestra familia.

28. ¿Por parte de su madre o de su padre?
    De los dos lados.

29. ¿Quién es su médico familiar?
    Es la Dra. Sánchez.

30. ¿Tiene enfermedades crónicas?
    Pues la diabetes y la presión alta.

31. ¿Desde cuándo las ha tenido?
    Desde hace 3 (tres) años.

32. Firme por favor en la pantalla.

Gracias. La receta va a estar lista pronto. ¿Va a pagar en efectivo, con tarjeta de crédito o con cheque?
Con mi tarjeta de débito.

Bien, pase a la caja, por favor.
Sí, claro.

Espere un momento. La farmacéutica le va a explicar cómo va a usar las medicinas.
Ah bueno. Muchas gracias.

Audio dialogue

PATIENT: *Hello, good morning. My name is Sonia Ramos. I have come to pick up the medicines for my mother, Lupita Salazar. Are they ready?*

TECHNICIAN: Let me see. One moment, please. When did you bring the prescription?

PATIENT: *She called yesterday. They are her medications for diabetes and blood pressure.*

TECHNICIAN: No, we couldn't fill them because we lack information. I need to ask you (make) some questions.

PATIENT: *That's fine.*

1. Today is September 16, 2008.

2. What is the complete name of your mother?
   It is Lupita Salazar Diego.

3. What is her last name (paternal)?
   It is Salazar.

4. What is her date of birth?
   January 6, 1942.

5. How old is she?
   She has 66 years.

6. What is her address?
   1328 López Anderson Avenue.

7. In what city and state?
   From here, El Paso, Texas.

8. What is her Zip code?
   79902.

9. What is her telephone number? Her cell? Her e-mail address?
   6-11-24-69. She doesn't have a cell phone or e-mail.

10. What is her occupation or profession?
    She is retired.

11. What is her marital status?
    She is married.

12. What is the name of her spouse or caretaker?
    My father, Ignacio Diego.

    Then her last name is Salazar or Diego?
    It is Diego.

13. Whom can we call in an emergency?
    Me, Sonia Ramos.

14. Once again, what is your relationship?
    I am her daughter.

15. What is your phone number?
    2-56-28-39.

16. What is the Social Security number of your mother?
    123-45-67-89.

17. What is her health insurance company?
    Medicare.

18. What is her (medication) policy number?
    It is the same as her Social Security.

19. Is your mother allergic to any medications?
    To penicillin and sulfa.

20. Is she a smoker?
    No.

21. What medications does she currently take?
    I think (that) lisinopril and metformin.

22. What is the dose? How often does she take them?
    (Of) 10 milligrams (mg) and (of) 500 mg. She takes her medications once a day.

23. What are they for?
    To control her blood pressure and diabetes.

24. What nonprescription medication does she take?
    Aspirin (of) 81 mg.

25. What herbal (natural) remedies does she take?
    Chamomile tea.

26. What vaccines has she received as an adult? Against influenza? Pneumonia? Tetanus?
    I took her to another pharmacy for a vaccine against influenza in October.

27. Does she have any risks for diseases in her family?
    Well, there are many people who have diabetes in our family.

28. From the side of her mother or her father?
    From both sides.

29. Who is her family doctor?
    It is Dr. Sánchez (female).

30. Does she have chronic diseases?
    Well, diabetes and high blood pressure.

31. How long has she had them?
    For (since) 3 years.

32. Sign on the screen, please.

Thank you. The prescription is going to be ready soon. Are you going to pay in cash, with a credit card, or with a check?
With my debit card.

Good, go to the cashier, please.
Of course.

Wait a moment. The pharmacist (female) is going to explain (to you) how she (your mother) is going to use the medicines.
All right. Thank you very much.

▮ *Vocabulario para la farmacia* / *Pharmacy vocabulary*

Verbos / Verbs		Presente / Present tense		
		Yo	Él, ella, usted	Mandato
abrir	to open	abro	abre	Abra
afectar(se)	to affect	afecto, me afecta	afecta, le afecta	Afecte
ayudar	to help	ayudo	ayuda	Ayude
caducar	to expire	—	caduca	Caduque
cargar	to charge	cargo	carga	Cargue
confirmar	to confirm	confirmo	confirma	Confirme
decir	to tell	digo	dice	Diga, Dígame
disculpar	to excuse, to be sorry	disculpo	disculpa	Disculpe, Discúlpeme
entregar	to deliver	entrego	entrega	Entregue
esperar	to wait, to hope	espero	espera	Espere
estar	to be (temporary)	estoy	está	Esté
evitar	to avoid, to prevent	evito	evita	Evite
explicar	to explain	explico	explica	Explique, Explíqueme
ir	to go	voy	va	Vaya
mandar	to send	mando	manda	Mande, Mándemelo(s)
necesitar	to need	necesito	necesita	Necesite
olvidar	to forget	olvido, se me olvida	olvida, se le olvida	Olvide, Olvídelo
pedir	to order	pido	pide	Pida
poder	to be able to (can)	puedo	puede	Pueda
preguntar	to ask	pregunto	pregunta	Pregunte
querer	to want	quiero	quiere	Quiera
recoger	to pick up	recojo	recoje	Recoja
recomendar	to recommend	recomiendo	recomienda	Recomiende
regresar	to return	regreso	regresa	Regrese
resurtir	to refill	resurto	resurte	Resurta
seguir	to follow	sigo	sigue	Siga
ser	to be (permanent)	soy	es	Sea
surtir	to fill (an order)	surto	surte	Surta
tener	to have	tengo	tiene	Tenga
tomar	to take	tomo	toma	Tome
usar	to use	uso	usa	Use
vencer(se)	to expire	—	se vence	Se venza

Sustantivos / Nouns

el artículo	item	la caja (la registradora)	cash register	la cola	line (queue)
la basura	trash	el cambio	change (coins)	la computadora	computer
la bolsa	bag	los centavos	cents	el cupón	coupon
la caducidad	expiration	el cesto de la basura	trash can	el dinero	money
		el cheque	check	el efectivo	cash

la fecha de caducidad (vencimiento)	expiration date				

Los lugares en la farmacia / Places in the pharmacy

Adjetivos / Adjectives

la fecha de caducidad (vencimiento) — expiration date

la licencia de manejar (conducir) — driver's license

la línea — line

el mostrador — counter

el precio — price

el producto — product

el recibo — receipt

el reembolso — refund

la señal — sign

la tarjeta de crédito — credit card

la tarjeta de seguro — insurance card

el timbre (la campanilla) — bell

el vencimiento — expiration

el ascensor, el elevador — elevator

el baño — bathroom

el bebedero — water fountain

la caja registradora, la caja — cashier's desk

el cajón — drawer

el cuarto — room

el estacionamiento — parking lot

el estante — rack, stand

el mostrador — counter

la oficina — office

la pared — wall

el pasillo — aisle

la puerta — door

la silla — chair

el suelo, el piso — floor

la ventana — window

barato(a) — inexpensive

caro(a) — expensive

correcto(a) — correct

equivocado(a) — wrong, mistaken

ocupado(a) — busy

Frases cortas / Short phrases

Debe formarse en la fila (haga fila) — Get in line

En especial (en oferta) — On sale

Entregamos a domicilio — We deliver

Estamos para servirle — At your service

Siga las instrucciones al pie de la letra — Follow the directions to the letter

¿Prefiere pagar en efectivo, con cheque o tarjeta de crédito? — Do you prefer to pay in cash, by check, or with a credit card?

▓ *Presentaciones de los medicamentos y otros productos / Formulations of medications and other products*

el aerosol, el espray — spray (nasal, topical)

la alimentación por sonda — enteral feeding

la ampolleta — ampule

el anestésico — anesthetic

el antibacteriano — antibacterial

la botella — bottle

la cápsula — capsule

el champú — shampoo

el chicle — gum (chewing)

la crema — cream, lotion

el desodorante — deodorant

la ducha femenina — feminine douche

la emulsión — emulsion

el enema — enema

la formulación — formulation (chemical)

el frasco — bottle

el frasco ámpula — vial

el gel — gel

las gotas — drops

el gotero — dropper

el inhalador — inhaler (nasal, oral)

la inyección intramuscular — intramuscular injection

la inyección intravenosa — intravenous injection

la inyección subcutánea — subcutaneous injection

el jabón — soap

el jarabe — syrup

la loción — clear solutions (e.g., astringents, perfume)

el óvulo vaginal — vaginal suppository

el parche — patch

la pastilla — pill

la perla — soft gel capsule

la píldora — very small round pills or "the pill" (contraceptive)

el polvo — medicinal powder (often oral)

la pomada — ointment

la presentación — formulation (packaged)

el purgante — purgative

la solución — solution

el suero — intravenous mixtures

el suero oral — electrolyte replacement (e.g., Pedialyte®)

el supositorio — suppository (rectal or vaginal)

la suspensión — suspension

la suspensión coloide — colloidal suspension

la tableta — tablet

el talco — powder (skin)

los toques — medication for mouth that is applied in "touches"

el trocisco — troche

el ungüento — cream, ointment

◼ *Las etiquetas para los productos* / *Auxiliary product labels*

Tómelo(la) con comida o leche	Take with food or milk
Tómelo(la) con mucha agua	Take with lots of water
Evite tomarlo(la) con calcio, hierro o productos lácteos	Avoid taking with calcium, iron, or milk products
No tome alcohol mientras toma la medicina.	Do not take with alcohol
Refrigérelo(la) por _____ días	Refrigerate (it) for _____ days
Evite el sol	Avoid the sun
Agítelo(la) bien	Shake (it) well
Sólo para uso externo	For external use only
Sólo para uso nasal	For nasal use only
Sólo para uso vaginal	For vaginal use only
Sólo para uso rectal	For rectal use only
Sólo para los ojos	For the eyes only
Sólo para los oídos	For the ears only
Evite usarlo si está embarazada o amamantando	Avoid using (it) if pregnant or breast-feeding
Puede causar mareo	May cause dizziness
Puede causar sueño	May cause drowsiness
Puede causar insomnio	May cause insomnia
No maneje mientras tome esta medicina	Do not drive while taking this medicine
Mantenga este medicamento fuera del alcance de los niños.	Keep this medication out of reach of children.

◼ *Unidades de medida* / *Units of measurement*

el centímetro	centimeter
el cuarto de galón	quart
la cuchara	tablespoon
la cucharada	tablespoonful
la cucharita	teaspoon
la cucharadita	teaspoonful
la(s) dosis	dose(s)
el grado centígrado	Centigrade
el grado fahrenheit	Fahrenheit
el galón	gallon
la gota	drop
el gramo	gram
el kilogramo	kilogram
la libra	pound
el litro	liter
el metro	meter
el miligramo	milligram
el mililitro	milliliter
la onza	ounce
el pie (los pies)	foot (feet)
la pinta	pint
la pulgada	inch
la taza	cup
la unidad	unit
el vaso	glass

Conversiones / Conversions

1 galón	3800 mL, 3.8 L	128 fl oz
0.26 galones	1 L	—
1 cuarto de galón*	960 mL	32 fl oz
1 pinta	480 mL	16 fl oz
1 taza	240 mL	8 fl oz
1 cucharada	15 mL	—
1 cucharadita	5 mL	—
3.28 pies (ft)	1 m	
1 pie (ft)	30.5 cm, 0.305 m	
1 pulgada (in)	2.54 cm	
0.39 pulgadas (in)	1 cm	
2.2 libras (lbs)	1 kg	
1 libra (lb)	0.45 kg	

*1 quart is about 1 liter.

Kilogramos	Libras
5 kg	11 lbs
10 kg	22 lbs
20 kg	44 lbs
30 kg	66 lbs
40 kg	88 lbs
50 kg	110 lbs
60 kg	132 lbs
70 kg	154 lbs
80 kg	176 lbs
90 kg	198 lbs
100 kg	220 lbs

Pies(') / pulgadas(") — Centímetros

Pies(') / pulgadas(")	Centímetros
2' (24")	61* cm
2' 6" (30")	76 cm
3' (36")	91.5 cm
3' 6" (42")	106.5 cm
4' (48")	122 cm
4' 6" (54")	137 cm
5' (60")	152.5 cm
5' 1" (61")	155 cm
5' 2" (62")	157.5 cm
5' 3" (63")	160 cm
5' 4" (64")	162.5 cm
5' 5" (65")	165 cm
5' 6" (66")	167.5 cm
5' 7" (67")	170 cm
5' 8" (68")	172.5 cm
5' 9" (69")	175 cm
5' 10" (70")	178 cm
5' 11" (71")	180.5 cm
6' (72")	183 cm
6' 1" (73")	185.5 cm
6' 2" (74")	188 cm
6' 3" (75")	190.5 cm

*Rounded to nearest 0.5 cm.

▇ *Las partes del cuerpo humano* / *The parts of the human body*
De la cabeza a los pies / Head to toe

la cabeza	head	la palma	palm	los oídos	ears (inner)
la cara	face	el dorso de la mano	back of the hand	la boca	mouth
el cuello	neck			los dientes	teeth
la nuca	nape	**La pierna**	**Leg**	las encías	gums
el hombro	shoulder	el muslo	thigh	la lengua	tongue
el pecho	chest	la rodilla	knee	los labios	lips
el seno, el pecho	breast	la pantorrilla	calf	la barbilla, el	chin
el pezón	nipple	el tobillo	ankle	mentón	
la costilla	rib	el pie	foot		
el abdomen	abdomen	el talón	heel	**Los órganos**	
el estómago	stomach	los dedos del pie	toes	**principales**	**Principal organs**
el ombligo	navel	la planta del pie	sole	el cerebro	brain
la cintura	waist			el pulmón	lung(s)
la espalda	back	**La cabeza**	**Head**	(los pulmones)	
la cadera	hip	el cabello, el pelo	hair	el corazón	heart
las nalgas, los glúteos,	buttocks	la frente	forehead	el estómago	stomach
las asentaderas		las sienes	temples	el hígado	liver
las pompis (euphemism)	buttocks	las cejas	eyebrows	el páncreas	pancreas
		los párpados	eyelids	el riñón (los	kidney(s)
		las pestañas	eyelashes	riñones)	
El brazo	**Arm**	los ojos	eyes	el intestino (los	intestine (bowels)
el antebrazo	forearm	las mejillas	cheeks	intestinos)	
el codo	elbow	la nariz	nose	el intestino grueso	large intestine
la mano	hand	las fosas, las	nostrils	el intestino	small intestine
los dedos	fingers	ventanas nasales		delgado	
la muñeca	wrist	las orejas	ears (outer)	la vesícula biliar	gallbladder

▇ *Las preguntas fundamentales* / *Prime questions*[1]

En el consultorio

FARMACÉUTICO(A): Esta medicina es aspirina.
¿Para qué es esta medicina?

PACIENTE: *No lo sé.*

FARMACÉUTICO(A): Esta medicina es para el corazón.

PACIENTE: *¡Ah es cierto! Me dijo la doctora que tomara aspirina para el corazón.*

FARMACÉUTICO(A): ¿Cómo va a tomar esta medicina?

PACIENTE: *Pues creo que dos o tres veces al día.*

FARMACÉUTICO(A): No exactamente. Usted debe tomar sólo 1 pastilla diariamente con comida. Cada pastilla es de 81 mg.
¿Me puede decir cuáles son los efectos secundarios de esta medicina?

PACIENTE: *¡Ay! Pues, no me acuerdo.*

FARMACÉUTICO(A): La aspirina le puede afectar el estómago. Por eso, debe tomarla con comida.
Ahora, quiero estar seguro(a) de que no olvidé nada.
Por favor explíqueme cómo va a tomar esta medicina.

PACIENTE: *Voy a tomar 1 aspirina solamente una vez al día con comida.*

In the counseling room

PHARMACIST: This medicine is aspirin.
What is this medication for?

PATIENT: *I don't know.*

PHARMACIST: This medicine is for your heart.

PATIENT: *Yes, that's true! The doctor told me that I should take aspirin for my heart.*

PHARMACIST: How are you going to take this medicine?

PATIENT: *Well, I believe two or three times a day.*

PHARMACIST: Not exactly. You must take only 1 pill daily with food. Each pill has 81 mg.
Can you tell me, what are the side effects of the medicine?

PATIENT: *Oh! I don't remember.*

PHARMACIST: Aspirin may affect your stomach. That is why you must take it with food.
Now, I want to be certain that I didn't forget anything. Please explain to me how you are going to take this medicine.

PATIENT: *I am going to take only 1 aspirin once a day with food.*

Medicamentos que no requieren receta médica / Nonprescription medications

1. ¿Para qué es esta medicina?
   What is this medicine for?

2. ¿Cómo va a tomar/usar esta medicina?
   How are you going to take/use this medicine?

3. ¿Cuáles son los efectos secundarios?
   What are the side effects?

4. Ahora, quiero estar seguro(a) de que no olvidé nada.
   Now, I want to make sure I didn't forget anything.

   Por favor, dígame cuáles son las instrucciones para tomar/usar esta medicina.
   Please, tell me what are the directions to take/use this medicine.

Nuevos medicamentos recetados / New prescriptions

1. ¿Para qué le dijo el doctor (la doctora) que era esta medicina?
   What did the doctor tell you the medicine was for?

2. ¿Cómo le dijo el doctor (la doctora) que tomara esta medicina?
   How did the doctor tell you to take the medicine?

3. ¿Qué le dijo el doctor (la doctora) que le podía pasar con esta medicina?
   What did the doctor tell you to expect (that could happen to you) from this medicine?

4. Ahora, quiero estar seguro(a) de que no olvidé nada.
   Now, I want to make sure that I didn't leave anything out.

   Por favor, dígame cómo va a tomar esta medicina.
   Please tell me how you are going to take your (the) medicine.

Resurtido de medicamentos recetados / Refill prescriptions

1. ¿Para qué toma/usa esta medicina?
   What do you take/use this medicine for?

2. ¿Cómo está tomando/usando la medicina?
   How do you take/use (are you taking/using) the medicine?

3. ¿Qué problemas ha tenido con la medicina?
   What kind of problems are you having (have you had) with the medicine?

4. ¿Me puede mostrar cómo está tomando/usando la medicina?
   Can you show me how you are taking/using the medicine?

◼ *Frases y preguntas para clarificar* / Phrases and questions of clarification

¿Tiene alguna pregunta?	Do you have any questions?
No entendí.	I didn't understand.
¿Mande?, ¿Sí?	What?
Repita por favor. ¿Cómo dijo?	Repeat to me please. (command) What did you say?
Hábleme más despacio, por favor.	Tell me more slowly, please. (command)
Dígame cosa por cosa (poco a poquito).	Tell me once again (a little at a time). (command)
Muéstreme dónde le duele.	Show me where it hurts you. (command)
Escríbalo, por favor.	Write it down for me, please. (command)
Lo siento.	I am sorry.
Un momento, necesito ayuda.	Just a moment, I need some assistance.

■ *Contestando el teléfono* / Answering the telephone

FARMACÉUTICA:	¡Bueno! Farmacia Sánchez. Soy _____. ¿En qué le puedo ayudar?
CLIENTE:	*Disculpe. ¿Qué horarios tienen? ¿A qué hora abren la farmacia?*
LA FARMACÉUTICA:	La farmacia está abierta de lunes a sábado.
EL CLIENTE:	*Muy bien. ¿De qué horas a qué horas?*
LA FARMACÉUTICA:	La farmacia está abierta de las 9:00 de la mañana a las 7:00 de la tarde.
EL CLIENTE:	*¿Pueden surtir mi medicina para mañana?*
LA FARMACÉUTICA:	Por supuesto. ¿Cuáles son los medicamentos que quiere surtir?
EL CLIENTE:	*Necesito más albuterol y lisinopril. ¿Cuándo puedo recogerlos? o ¿Pueden mandarlos a mi casa?*
LA FARMACÉUTICA:	Si, podemos mandarlos. Pero quiero confirmar cuántas veces al día está tomando los medicamentos.
EL CLIENTE:	*Estoy usando el inhalador cuando es necesario. Y del lisinopril estoy tomando 1 pastilla cada mañana. Casi se me olvidaba —voy a salir de viaje. ¿Necesito evitar los rayos del sol?*
LA FARMACÉUTICA:	No, los medicamentos no van a afectar tanto su sensibilidad al sol. Pero es muy importante que siga las instrucciones al pie de la letra. ¿Tiene otra pregunta?
EL CLIENTE:	*Por ahora, no. Es muy amable. Gracias por su ayuda. Adiós.*
LA FARMACÉUTICA:	De nada, es un placer. Estamos para servirle.

PHARMACIST:	Hello! Sánchez Pharmacy. I am _____. How can I help you?
CUSTOMER:	*Excuse me. What is your schedule (do you have)? At what hour do you open the pharmacy?*
PHARMACIST:	The pharmacy is open from Monday to Saturday.
CUSTOMER:	*All right. At what time is the pharmacy open? (From what hour to what hour?)*
PHARMACIST:	The pharmacy is open from 9:00 in the morning to 7:00 in the afternoon.
CUSTOMER:	*Could you fill in my medicine for tomorrow?*
PHARMACIST:	Of course. What are the medications that you want to fill?
CUSTOMER:	*I need more albuterol and lisinopril. When can I pick them up? Or can you deliver them to my house?*
PHARMACIST:	Yes, we can deliver them. But I want to confirm how many times a day you are taking the medications.
CUSTOMER:	*I am using the inhaler when it is necessary. And the lisinopril, I am taking 1 pill each morning. I almost forgot—I am going on a trip. Do I need to avoid the sun (rays)?*
PHARMACIST:	No, the medications are not going to affect your sensitivity to the sun too much. But it is very important that you follow the directions very carefully. Do you have another question?
CUSTOMER:	*For now, no. You are very kind. Thank you for your help. Goodbye.*
PHARMACIST:	You are welcome (it is nothing); it's a pleasure. We are at your service.

REFERENCE

1. Gardner M, Boyce RW, Herrier RN. *Pharmacist–Patient Consultation Program PPCP-Unit I: An Interactive Approach to Verifying Patient Understanding.* New York: Pfizer Educational Services; 1990.

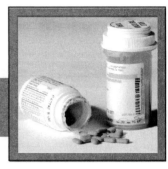

Analgésicos y antipiréticos
Analgesics and antipyretics

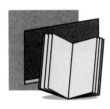

Lección 1   Dolores musculares
Lesson 1   Muscle pain

Verbos / Verbs		Presente / Present tense			
		Yo	Él, ella, usted	Mandato	Ejemplos
aliviar	to alleviate	alivio	alivia	Alivie	*La medicina **alivia** el dolor.*
aliviar(se)	to feel better	me alivio	se alivia	Alíviese	***Alíviese** pronto.*
calmar(se)	to relieve	se me calma	se le calma	Cálmese	*La reuma se **me calma** con el analgésico.*
					***Cálmese** por favor.*
cambiar	to change	cambio	cambia	Cambie	*¿El dolor **cambia**?*
					***Cambie** de medicina.*
caminar	to walk	camino	camina	Camine	*Yo **camino** todos los días.*
causar	to cause	causo	causa	No cause*	*¿Qué **causa** el problema?*
controlar	to control	controlo	controla	Controle	*¿Cómo **controla** el dolor?*
dar	to give	doy	da	Déme	***Déme** la receta, por favor.*
decir	to say	digo	dice	Dígame	***Dígame**, ¿dónde le duele?*
		le dije†	me dijo†		
describir	to describe	describo	describe	Describa	***Describa** el dolor.*
doler(se)	to hurt, to be in pain	me duele	le duele	—	*¿**Le duele** el pecho?*
		me duelen	le duelen		***Me dolió** mucho el brazo.*
		me dolió†	le dolió†		
dormir(se)	to sleep	me duermo	se duerme	Duérmase	*¿**Duerme** bien en la noche?*
empeorar	to worsen	empeoro	empeora	No empeore*	*¿Qué **empeora**?*
estar	to be (location, feeling)	estoy	está	Esté	***Estoy** en la farmacia.*
					***Esté** en la clínica a las 8:00 de la mañana.*

continued on p.14

Verbos / Verbs   Presente / Present tense

		Yo	Él, ella, usted	Mandato	Ejemplos
gustar	to like	me gusta me gustan	le gusta le gustan	—	¿*Le gusta* caminar? No *me gusta* la medicina.
haber (hay)	to have there is, there are	—	—	—	¿*Hay* más inflamación en las mañanas?
hacer	to do, to make	hago	hace	Haga Hágalo (*Do it*)	¿Qué *hace* para aliviar el dolor? *Haga* ejercicio todos los días.
mostrar	to show	muestro	muestra	Muestre Muéstreme	*Muéstreme* dónde le duele.
olvidar	to forget	olvido se me olvida	olvida se le olvida	No se le olvide (*Don't forget*)	No *se le olvide* tomar la medicina.
poder	to be able to (can)	puedo	puede	—	¿*Puede* dormir bien?
sentir sentir(se)	to feel to feel (oneself)	siento me siento	siente se siente	Sienta Siéntase	¿Cómo *se siente* hoy? *Me siento* mal.
ser	to be (permanent)	soy	es	Sea	*Soy* la farmacéutica. *Sea* persistente, tome la medicina siempre.
tener*	to have	tengo tuve† tenía†	tiene tuvo† tenía†	Tenga	¿*Tiene* dolor? ¡*Tenga* buen día!
tener que	to have to	tengo que	tiene que	—	*Tiene que* tomar el analgésico.
tomar	to take	tomo tomé†	toma tomó†	Tome Tómelo (*Take it*)	*Tome* la medicina con comida. *Tómelo* (el medicamento) sólo cuando sea necesario.

*This command is frequently used in the negative. †These verbs are often used in the past tenses, particularly by the patient.

Las partes del cuerpo /Parts of the body*

la articulación	joint
el brazo	arm
el cuello	neck
el cuerpo	body
los dedos de la mano	fingers
los dedos del pie	toes
la espalda	back
el hueso	bone
la mano	hand
el músculo	muscle
el pie	foot
la pierna	leg

Sustantivos / Nouns

la acidez	heartburn
el analgésico	analgesic
el bienestar	comfort, well-being
el calambre	cramp
la comida	food
el dolor	pain
el enrojecimiento	redness
la escala	rating scale
la incomodidad	discomfort
la inflamación	inflammation
la leche	milk

el malestar	discomfort
la molestia	discomfort
la náusea	nausea
la parte	part

Adjetivos / Adjectives

agudo(a)	sharp
caliente	hot
continuo(a)	continuous
dañino(a)	damaging
frío(a)	cold
fuerte	strong
hinchado(a)	swollen
igual	equal, same
incómodo(a)	uncomfortable
inflamado(a)	inflamed
intenso(a)	intense
leve	slight
ligero(a)	light (not heavy)
mejor	better
molesto(a)	bothersome
mucho(a)	a lot, much
muchísimo(a)	very much
peor	worse
persistente	persistent
sordo(a)	dull (pain)
tolerable	tolerable

Otras expresiones / Other expressions

ahora	now
ahora mismo	right now
ahorita	right now, in a few moments
Alíviese pronto	Get well soon
bien	well
cada	each, every
con	with
después	after, later
en otras palabras	in other words
es decir	that is to say
hacer ejercicio	to exercise
mal	bad
mire	look (to get attention)
muy	very
o	or
o sea	in other words
poco (a)	little
por eso	for that reason
si es necesario	if needed
siempre	always
sin	without
va y viene	comes and goes
y	and

*When one is speaking about a body part in Spanish, the definite article (el, la, los, las) is often used instead of the possessive pronoun (e.g., mi, su).

Preguntas[1]
1. ¿Dónde le duele? ¿En qué partes del cuerpo?
2. ¿Desde cuándo tiene el dolor?
3. ¿Qué tan seguido tiene el dolor? ¿Qué tan frecuente siente el dolor?
4. Describa el dolor. ¿Es agudo o sordo? ¿Es como reuma, continuo? ¿Es muy intenso?
5. ¿Qué le empeora el dolor? ¿Qué le mejora el dolor? ¿Qué le calma el dolor?
6. ¿Hay inflamación o enrojecimiento? ¿Tiene dolor en las articulaciones? ¿Tiene calambres?
7. Piense en una escala de cero al diez para describir el dolor.[2]
   El cero representa poco o nada de dolor, es decir es tolerable.
   El diez representa muchísimo dolor, un dolor muy fuerte.
   Ahora, usted describa el dolor.
8. ¿El dolor es igual o cambia? ¿Va y viene?
9. ¿Cuándo es peor el dolor? ¿En las noches? ¿Cuando hace ejercicio?
10. ¿Toma algún medicamento para controlar o aliviar el dolor?

Recomendaciones
1. Esta medicina es ibuprofeno de 200 (dos cientos) mg (miligramos).
2. Esta medicina le va a calmar el dolor.
3. Tome 1 (una) o 2 (dos) pastillas cada 6 (seis) a 8 (ocho) horas, sólo si tiene dolor.
4. Tómela con comida o con leche.

Efectos secundarios (molestias)
Puede causarle acidez, dolor de estómago, o náuseas ligeras.

Las preguntas fundamentales[3]
1. ¿Para qué es esta medicina?
2. ¿Cómo va a usar esta medicina?
3. ¿Cuáles son los efectos secundarios?
4. Quiero confirmar que no olvidé nada. Ahora me puede explicar cómo va a usar esta medicina.

Questions for the patient[1]*

1. Where does it hurt you? In what parts of the body?
2. How long have you had the pain?
3. How often do you have the pain? How frequently do you feel the pain?
4. Describe the pain. Is it sharp or dull? Is it like a dull pain, continuous? Is it intense?
5. What worsens the pain? What improves the pain? What relieves the pain?
6. Is there inflammation or redness? Do you have pain in your joints? Do you have cramps?
7. Think of a scale between (from) zero to ten to describe the pain.[2]
   Zero represents very little or no (nothing of) pain, that is to say it is tolerable.
   Ten represents a lot of pain, a very strong pain.
   Now, describe the pain.
8. Is the pain equal or does it change? Does it come and go?
9. When is the pain worse? At night? When you exercise?
10. Do you take any medication to control or alleviate the pain?

Recommendations

1. This medicine is ibuprofen 200 mg (milligrams).
2. It is going to relieve your pain.
3. Take 1 or 2 pills every 6 to 8 hours, only if you have pain.
4. Take it with food or milk.

Side effects

It can cause heartburn, stomach pain, or light nausea.

Prime questions[3]

1. What is this medication for?
2. How are you going to use this medication?
3. What are the side effects?
4. I want to make sure that I didn't forget anything. Now, can you explain to me how you are going to use this medicine?

---

*Not all of the English translations throughout the book are written in standard English. Rather, they are a close literal translation from Spanish. This more literal translation can be a helpful teaching tool that allows the student to better understand grammatical rules and the arrangement of words (syntax) in the Spanish language.

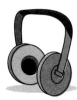

Diálogos para el audio

FARMACÉUTICA: Buenas tardes. Soy la Dra. Jones, su farmacéutica. ¿Cómo le puedo ayudar?

PACIENTE: *Mucho gusto, doctora. Pues, mire, no me siento bien, me duele todo el cuerpo. Tengo un dolor muy fuerte. No puedo caminar bien por el dolor. ¿Qué puedo tomar? No tengo receta médica.*

FARMACÉUTICA: Entiendo, primero tengo algunas preguntas para usted.

Preguntas[1]

1. ¿Dónde le duele? ¿En qué partes del cuerpo?
   Me duelen las piernas y también la espalda.

2. ¿Desde cuándo tiene dolor?
   Desde hace 2 días.

3. ¿Qué tan seguido tiene el dolor? ¿Qué tan frecuente siente el dolor?
   Siento el dolor más fuerte en las mañanas.

4. Describa el dolor. ¿Es agudo o sordo? ¿Es como reuma, continuo? ¿Es muy intenso?
   Es sordo.

5. ¿Qué le empeora el dolor? ¿Qué le mejora el dolor? ¿Qué le calma el dolor?
   Cuando cambio de posición, siento mucho dolor e incomodidad.

6. ¿Hay inflamación o enrojecimiento? ¿Tiene dolor en las articulaciones? ¿Tiene calambres?
   Hay poquito enrojecimiento. No tengo dolor en las articulaciones ni calambres.

7. Lo siento. Piense en una escala de cero al diez para describir el dolor.[2]
   El cero representa poco o nada de dolor, es decir es tolerable.
   El diez representa muchísimo dolor, un dolor muy fuerte.
   Ahora, usted describa el dolor.
   Mi dolor es del número tres, más o menos.

8. ¿El dolor es igual o cambia? ¿Va y viene?
   Es igual. Es más o menos constante.

9. ¿Cuándo es peor el dolor? ¿En las noches? ¿Cuando hace ejercicio o camina?
   Es peor cuando hago ejercicio por más de 2 horas.

10. ¿Toma algún medicamento para controlar o aliviar el dolor?
    No, ahora, no estoy tomando nada.

Recomendaciones

1. Esta medicina es ibuprofeno de 200 (doscientos) mg.
2. Esta medicina le va a calmar el dolor.
3. Tome 1 o 2 pastillas cada 6 (seis) a 8 (ocho) horas, sólo si tiene dolor.
4. Tómela con comida o con leche.

Efectos secundarios (molestias)

Esta medicina puede causarle acidez, dolor de estómago o náuseas ligeras.

Las preguntas fundamentales[3]

1. ¿Para qué es esta medicina?
   Esta medicina se llama ibuprofeno de 200 mg. Es para aliviar el dolor muscular.

2. ¿Cómo va a usar esta medicina?
   Voy a tomar de 1 o 2 pastillas cada 6 a 8 horas, sólo si tengo dolor. Debo tomar el ibuprofeno con leche o con comida para evitar las molestias del estómago.

3. ¿Cuáles son los efectos secundarios?
   El ibuprofeno puede causarme acidez, dolor de estómago o náuseas ligeras.

4. Quiero confirmar que no olvidé nada. Ahora, usted me puede explicar cómo va a usar esta medicina.
   Sí. Voy a tomar de 1 o 2 pastillas cada 6 a 8 horas con leche o con comida para aliviar el dolor muscular de la espalda o de las piernas. Debo tomar las pastillas solamente si tengo dolor fuerte. La medicina se llama ibuprofeno y no requiere receta médica. Cada pastilla es de 200 mg.

Muy bien. Ojalá que se sienta mejor. Hasta luego.

Gracias. Hasta luego.

◼ *Audio dialogues*

PHARMACIST: Good afternoon. I am Dr. Jones, your pharmacist. How can I help you?

PATIENT: *Nice to meet you, Doctor. Well, you see, I do not feel very well, my body aches all over. The pain hurts a lot. I can't walk well because of the pain. What can I take? I do not have a prescription.*

PHARMACIST: I understand, but first I have a few questions for you.

Questions[1]

1. Where does it hurt? In what parts of the body?
   My legs and also my back hurt.

2. How long have you had the pain?
   For 2 days.

3. How often do you have the pain? How frequently do you feel the pain?
   The pain is worst in the mornings.

4. Describe the pain. Is it sharp or dull? Is it like a dull pain, continuous? Is it intense?
   It's a dull pain.

5. What worsens the pain? What improves the pain? What relieves the pain?
   When I change positions I feel a lot of pain and discomfort.

6. Is there inflammation or redness? Do you have pain in your joints? Do you have cramps?
   There is some redness. I don't have pain in my joints or cramps.

7. I'm sorry. Think of a scale between (from) zero to ten to describe the pain.[2]
   Zero represents (is) very little or no (nothing of) pain, that is to say it is tolerable.
   Ten represents a lot of pain, a very strong pain.
   Now, describe the pain.
   My pain is at number three, more or less.

8. Is the pain equal, or does it change? Does it come and go?
   It's about the same. It's more or less constant.

9. When is the pain worse? At night? When you exercise or walk?
   It is worse when I exercise for more than 2 hours.

10. Do you use some medication to control or alleviate the pain?
    No, I'm not taking anything now.

Recommendations

1. This medicine is ibuprofen 200 mg.
2. It is going to relieve your pain.
3. Take 1 or 2 pills every 6 to 8 hours, only if you have pain.
4. Take it with food or milk.

Side effects

This medicine can cause heartburn, stomach pain, or light nausea.

Prime questions[3]

1. What is this medication for?
   This medication is ibuprofen 200 mg. It is to alleviate muscle pain.

2. How are you going to use this medication?
   I am going to take 1 or 2 pills every 6 to 8 hours only if I have pain. I should take this medicine with food or milk to avoid stomach discomfort.

3. What are the side effects?
   Ibuprofen may cause heartburn, stomach pain, or light nausea.

4. I want to make sure that I didn't forget anything. Now, can you explain to me how you are going to use this medicine?
   Yes. I am going to take 1 or 2 pills every 6 to 8 hours with milk or food to relieve the muscle pain in my (of the) back or legs. I should take the pills only if I have a strong pain. The medicine is called ibuprofen and doesn't require a prescription. Each pill is 200 mg.

Very good. I hope that you feel better. See you later.

Thank you. See you later.

De la cultura / About the culture

1. In some Hispanic communities, patients may say "**me duelen los huesos,**" which translates literally to "my bones hurt." These patients may actually be referring to their muscles. The term "**huesos**" can refer to the body in general.

2. The verb "**calmar(se)**" can be used to describe physical pain and emotional distress. For example, "**Cálmese**" can mean "Relax" or "Calm down."

3. "**Reuma**" may be used to refer to a dull pain found mainly in the legs and arms. Literally, it can be translated to "rheumatism." However, patients do not have to have this diagnosis to make the complaint "**Tengo reumas en las piernas.**"

4. In some Hispanic cultures, "**ahorita**" may mean "in a few moments" or "when I can get around to it," contradicting the literal translation "right now." For "at this very moment," the expression is "**ahora mismo.**"

5. Some patients may not understand "**efectos secundarios,**" in which case "**molestias**" may be used.

Apuntes de gramática / Grammar notes

Grammar topics in this section include the following:

Verbs with indirect object pronouns	Example: (doler) (to hurt)	¿<u>Le duelen</u> las piernas? Do your legs <u>hurt you</u>?
Reflexive verbs	Example: (sentirse) (to feel [oneself])	<u>Me siento</u> mejor ahora. <u>I feel (myself)</u> better now.
Future progressive	Example: (ir + a + infinitive) (going + to + infinitive)	<u>Voy a tomar</u> la medicina. <u>I am going to take</u> the medicine.
Compound verbs	Example: (necesitar + infinitive) (to need to + infinitive)	<u>Necesito tomar</u> esta medicina. <u>I need to take</u> this medicine.
Commands (mandatos)	Example: (dar) (to give)	<u>Déme</u> la receta. <u>Give</u> me the prescription.

Ejercicios / Exercises

I. Llene los espacios en blanco con la palabra o expresión apropiada. (Fill in the blanks with the appropriate word or expression.)

1. *Paciente:* Buenas tardes, doctor, tengo un _____ muy fuerte en las piernas. ¿Qué medicina me (poder / aliviar) _____ _____ este dolor?

2. **Farmacéutico:** ¿Cómo es el dolor, Sra. García? ¿Es _____, _____ o _____?

3. *Paciente:* Bueno, por las noches (dormir) _____ sin molestias. Pero durante el día, el dolor es muy _____. Cuando (hacer) _____ ejercicio (sentirse) ____ _____ muy mal. El dolor es _____ y no puedo caminar fácilmente.

4. **Farmacéutico:** ¿Le dan _____?

5. *Paciente:* No sé. Pero me (doler) _____ mucho las piernas y veo que (estar / inflamar) _____. Mírelas.

II. Relacione las siguientes palabras con los sinónimos o antónimos correctos. (Match the words with their correct synonym or antonym.)

Sinónimos

____1. continuo   a. hinchado
____2. ligera   b. molestias
____3. inflamado   c. persistente
____4. efectos secundarios   d. leve

Antónimos

____1. peor   a. sordo
____2. agudo   b. bienestar
____3. dolor   c. mejor
____4. con   d. frío
____5. caliente   e. sin

III. Haga una pregunta para cada respuesta. (Write a question for each answer.)

1. ¿_____?
   Me siento mal.

2. ¿_____?
   Me duele la espalda.

3. ¿_____?
   Tomo paracetamol (un analgésico) cada noche.

4. ¿_____?
   Los tengo inflamados después de caminar.

5. ¿_____?
   Puede causarme náusea ligera o malestar en el estómago. Por eso, tengo que tomarla con comida o leche.

IV. Escriba una oración con las siguientes palabras. (Write a sentence using the following words.)

1. piernas / doler / noches

2. pastilla / causar / molestia / náusea / acidez

3. músculo / inflamarse / ejercicio

4. dolor / describir / sordo / persistente

V. Busque en el Internet un sitio en español y escriba un párrafo sobre uno de los siguientes temas. (Look up an Internet site in Spanish and write a paragraph about one of the following topics.)

1. paracetamol

2. ibuprofeno

3. dolores musculares

4. analgésicos

REFERENCES

1. Wright E. Musculoskeletal injuries and disorders. In: Berardi RR, Kroon LA, McDermott JH, et al., eds. *Handbook of Nonprescription Drugs.* 15th ed. Washington, DC: American Pharmacists Association; 2006:109–31.
2. Seidel HM, Gall JW, Dains JE, et al. *Mosby's Guide to Physical Examination, 4th Ed.* St. Louis, Mo: Mosby, Inc 1999:908–10.
3. Gardner M, Boyce RW, Herrier RN. *Pharmacist–Patient Consultation Program PPCP-Unit I: An Interactive Approach to Verifying Patient Understanding.* New York: Pfizer Educational Services; 1991.

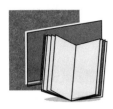

Lección 2   Fiebre
Lesson 2   Fever

Verbos / Verbs   Presente / Present tense

		Yo	Él, ella, usted	Mandato	Ejemplos
afectar	to affect	me afecta	le afecta	Afecte	*La medicina le afecta el estómago.*
agitar	to shake	agito	agita	Agite	*Agite la suspensión antes de tomarla.*
arder(se)	to burn	me arde	le arde	Arda	*El estómago me arde con la medicina.*
contener	to contain	contengo	contiene	Contenga	*La suspensión contiene acetaminofén.*
haber	to have	he	ha	—	*He tenido fiebre.*
ir	to go	voy	va	Vaya	*Vaya con el doctor.*
llamar (se)	to name, to call	llamo me llamo	llama se llama	Llame	*¿Cómo se llama?* *Llame a la clínica.*
llevar	to take, to carry	llevo	lleva	Lleve	*Lleve su receta a la farmacia.*
llorar	to cry	lloro	llora	No llore*	*No llore tanto, cálmese.*
medir	to measure	mido	mide	Mida	*Mida la medicina.*
necesitar	to need	necesito	necesita	—	*Usted necesita un termómetro.*
repetir	to repeat, to belch	repito	repite	Repita	*Repita el número, por favor.*

*This command is frequently used in the negative.

Sustantivos / Nouns

el adulto, la adulta	adult
la botella	bottle
la calentura	fever
el comprimido	pill
la cuchara	tablespoon
la cucharada	tablespoonful
la cucharadita	teaspoonful
la cucharita	teaspoon
la edad	age
el elíxir	elixir
la febrícula	low-grade fever
la gota	drop
el gotero	dropperful
el grado	degree
el hijo, la hija	son, daughter
la infección	infection
el jarabe	syrup
la jeringa	syringe
el niño, la niña	boy, girl
el supositorio	suppository
la suspensión	suspension
la tableta	tablet
la temperatura	temperature
el termómetro	thermometer

Adjetivos / Adjectives

caliente	hot
confiable	safe, reliable
dañino(a)	harmful
efectivo(a)	effective
masticable	chewable
peligroso(a)	dangerous
plástico(a)	plastic
seguro(a)	safe (for use), sure (certain)

Termómetros / Thermometers

en la axila	axillary
debajo del brazo	under the arm(pit)
del oído	tympanic
oral	oral
rectal	rectal

Centígrado / Celsius	Fahrenheit
36°	96.8°
37°	**98.6°**
38°	100.4°
39°	102.2°
40°	104.0°

Otras expresiones / Other expressions

algo de calentura	some fever
antes de	before
la dosis exacta	exact dose
generalmente	generally
más de	more than [before a number]
para bebés	for infants
para niños	for children
pasar de	to be over
sabor a cereza	cherry flavored
sabor a frutas	fruit flavored
sabor a uva	grape flavored
también	too, also
usualmente	usually
Se siente caliente.	He or she feels hot to the touch.

Preguntas[1]

1. ¿Qué temperatura tiene su hijo(a)?
2. ¿Desde cuándo tiene fiebre?
3. ¿Ha tenido una temperatura que pase de 38 grados?
4. ¿Qué edad tiene el niño (la niña)?
5. ¿Le está dando un medicamento para la fiebre?
6. ¿Ha llevado a su hijo(a) con el (la) doctor(a)?
7. ¿Cuánto pesa el niño (la niña)?

Recomendaciones (para un niño de 7 años)[2]

1. Voy a darle una suspensión que se llama acetaminofén para su hijo. Contiene 160 (ciento sesenta) mg por cada cucharita.
2. Déle 2 cucharaditas* cada 4 a 6 horas si tiene temperatura.
3. Si no tiene una cucharita, puede medir la suspensión con una jeringa plástica de 10 mL (mililitros).
4. Agite muy bien la botella antes de darle la medicina. Asegúrese de que ha medido la cantidad exacta.

Dosis de acetaminofén para los bebés y los niños (~10–15 mg/kg/dosis)[2]

Edad	Dosis (mg)	160 mg / 5 mL	80 mg / 0.8 mL
0–3 meses	40	—	½ gotero (0.4 mL)
4–11 meses	80	—	1 gotero (0.8 mL)
1–2 años	120	—	1½ goteros (1.2 mL)
2–3 años	160	1 cucharita (5.0 mL)	2 goteros (1.6 mL)
4–5 años	240	1½ cucharitas (7.5 mL)	—
6–8 años	320	2 cucharitas (10.0 mL)	—
9–10 años	400	2½ cucharitas (12.5 mL)	—
11 años	480	1 cucharada* (15.0 mL)	—

Efectos secundarios (molestias)

1. Generalmente esta medicina es segura y efectiva.
2. Pero puede ser dañina al hígado si se toma en más cantidad de la necesaria o por más tiempo que el indicado.
3. No les dé a sus hijos(as) más de 2.6 (dos punto seis) gramos al día. No les dé más de 5 dosis al día.[2]
4. Toxicidad en adultos: Si toma más de 4 gramos al día le puede afectar el hígado.

Las preguntas fundamentales[3]

1. ¿Para qué es esta medicina?
2. ¿Cómo va a darle esta medicina a su hijo(a)?
3. ¿Cuáles son los efectos secundarios?
4. Quiero confirmar que no se me olvidó nada. Por favor, repita cómo va a darle esta medicina a su hijo(a).

---

*Cucharadita—teaspoon measurement; cucharita (1 teaspoon = 5 mL).
 Cucharada—tablespoon measurement; cuchara (1 tablespoon = 15 mL).

Questions[1]

1. What temperature does your son (daughter) have?
2. How long has he (she) had a fever?
3. Has he (she) had a temperature over 38°C?
4. How old is the boy (girl)?
5. Are you giving him (her) any medication for the fever?
6. Have you taken your son (daughter) to the doctor?
7. How much does the boy (girl) weigh?

Recommendations (for a 7-year-old boy)

1. I am going to give you an acetaminophen suspension for your son. It has 160 mg per teaspoon.
2. Give your child 2 teaspoonfuls every 4 to 6 hours if he has a fever.
3. If you don't have a teaspoon, you can measure the suspension in a plastic syringe with 10 mL (milliliters).
4. Shake the bottle very well before giving him the medicine. Make sure that you have measured the exact quantity.

Acetaminophen dosage for infants and children (~10–15 mg/kg/dose)[2]

Age	Dosage (mg)	160 mg / 5 mL	80 mg / 0.8 mL
0–3 months	40	—	½ dropperful (0.4 mL)
4–11 months	80	—	1 dropperful (0.8 mL)
1–2 years	120	—	1½ droppersful (1.2 mL)
2–3 years	160	1 teaspoon (5.0 mL)	2 droppersful (1.6 mL)
4–5 years	240	1½ teaspoons (7.5 mL)	—
6–8 years	320	2 teaspoons (10.0 mL)	—
9–10 years	400	2½ teaspoons (12.5 mL)	—
11 years	480	1 tablespoon (15.0 mL)	—

Side effects

1. This medicine is generally very safe and effective.
2. But it can be harmful to the liver if more than the recommended dosage is taken or for more time than indicated.
3. Do not give your children more than 2.6 grams per day. Do not give them more than 5 doses per day.
4. Adult toxicity: If you take more than 4 grams a day, it can affect your liver.

Prime questions[3]

1. What is this medication for?
2. How are you going to give this medication to your son (daughter)?
3. What are the side effects?
4. I want to make sure that I didn't forget anything. Please, can you repeat to me how you are going to give this medicine to your son (daughter)?

Diálogos para el audio

FARMACÉUTICO: Buenas noches. Soy el Dr. James Levín, su farmacéutico. ¿Cómo le puedo ayudar?

PACIENTE: *Buenas noches, Dr. Levin. Pues, creo que mi hija tiene algo de calentura. Esta tarde no quiso comer ni*
(PAPÁ) *tampoco jugar pero sí fue a la escuela. Y ahora es muy noche. No sé qué darle para que se sienta mejor.*
¿Qué me recomienda?

Preguntas[1]

1. ¿Qué temperatura tiene su hija?
   Le tomé la temperatura oral hace 2 horas. Tenía 37.8 grados.

2. ¿Desde cuándo tiene fiebre?
   Desde ayer en la noche tiene algo de calentura.

3. ¿Ha tenido una temperatura que pase de 38 grados?
   No, pero ahorita se siente más caliente.

4. ¿Qué edad tiene su niña?
   Tiene 7 años.

5. ¿Le está dando un medicamento para la fiebre?
   No, no le he dado nada.

6. ¿Ha llevado a su hija con el doctor?
   Sí, ayer fuimos con el doctor. Me recomendó una medicina para bajarle la fiebre. ¿Podemos comprarla sin receta?

   Sí, claro, no necesita receta médica.

7. ¿Cuánto pesa la niña?
   No estoy seguro. Tiene 7 años y creo que pesa como 30 kilos más o menos.

Recomendaciones

1. Voy a darle una suspensión que se llama acetaminofén para su hija. Contiene 160 (ciento sesenta) mg por cada cucharita.
2. Déle 2 cucharaditas cada 4 a 6 horas si tiene temperatura. La niña va a necesitar 320 mg o 10 mL de acetaminofén cada 4 a 6 horas. Ésta es la dosis exacta.
3. Si no tiene una cucharita también puede medir la suspensión con una jeringa plástica de 10 mL como ésta.
4. Agite muy bien la botella antes de medir y darle la medicina. Asegúrese de que ha medido la cantidad o dosis exacta y que ha esperado 4 a 6 horas antes de darle la siguiente dosis.

Efectos secundarios (molestias)

1. Generalmente esta medicina es segura y efectiva.
2. Puede ser dañina al hígado si se administra en mucha cantidad o por más tiempo que el indicado.
3. No le dé a su hija más de 2.6 (dos punto seis) gramos cada día. No le dé más de 5 dosis al día.

Las preguntas fundamentales[3]

1. ¿Para qué es esta medicina?
   Esta medicina se llama acetaminofén en suspensión. Es para bajar la temperatura cuando hay fiebre.

2. ¿Cómo va a darle esta medicina a su hija?
   Voy a darle 2 cucharitas o 10 mL cada 4 a 6 horas solamente si tiene calentura o tiene una temperatura más alta de 38 grados. Voy a medir la dosis con la jeringa de plástico.

3. ¿Cuáles son los efectos secundarios?
   No hay efectos secundarios, pero no debo darle demasiada medicina.

4. Quiero confirmar que no olvidé nada. Por favor, dígame, ¿cómo va a darle esta medicina a su hija?
   Esta medicina se llama acetaminofén en suspensión. Es para bajar la temperatura cuando hay fiebre. Voy a darle 2 cucharitas o 10 mL cada 4 a 6 horas solamente si tiene calentura. Voy a medir la dosis con la jeringa de plástico.

Muy bien. Espero que su hija se alivie muy pronto. Que le vaya muy bien.

Muchas gracias, doctor. Adiós.

Audio dialogues

PHARMACIST: Good evening. I am Dr. James Levin, your pharmacist. How can I help you?

PATIENT: *Good evening, Dr. Levin. Well, I think that my daughter is running a slight fever. This afternoon she did not want to eat or*
(FATHER) *play, but she did go to school. Now it is late. I do not know what to give her to feel better. What do you recommend?*

Questions[1]

1. What temperature does your daughter have?
   I took her temperature by mouth about 2 hours ago. She had a temperature of 37.8 degrees.

2. How long has she had a fever?
   Since last night she has some fever.

3. Has she had a temperature over 38 degrees?
   No, but right now she feels slightly warmer.

4. How old is your daughter?
   My daughter is 7 years old.

5. Are you giving her any medication for the fever?
   No, I haven't given her anything.

6. Have you taken your daughter to the doctor?
   Yes. Yesterday, we went to the doctor. He recommended that I give her medicine to reduce the fever. Can we buy this medicine without a prescription?

   Yes. You don't need a prescription for this medicine.

7. How much does your daughter weigh?
   I am not sure. She is 7 years old and I believe that she weighs about 30 kilograms more or less.

Recommendations

1. I am going to give you an acetaminophen suspension for your daughter. It has 160 mg per teaspoon.
2. Give your daughter 2 teaspoonfuls every 4 to 6 hours if she has fever. Your daughter is going to need to take 320 mg or 10 mL (milliliters) of acetaminophen every 4 to 6 hours to reduce the fever. This is the exact dosage.
3. If you don't have a teaspoon, you can measure the suspension in a plastic syringe with 10 mL, like this one.
4. Shake the bottle very well before measuring and giving the medicine to your child. Make sure that you have measured the exact

quantity of the medicine and that you have waited 4 to 6 hours before giving to her the next dose.

Side effects

1. This medicine is generally very safe and effective.
2. It can be harmful to the liver if too much is taken or for more time than indicated.
3. Do not give her more than 2.6 grams per day. Do not give her more than 5 doses a day.

Fundamental questions

1. What is this medication for?
   This medicine is an acetaminophen suspension. This medicine will reduce her fever.

2. How are you going to give this medication to your daughter?
   I am going to give her 2 teaspoonfuls or 10 mL every 4 to 6 hours only if she has a fever or if she has a temperature more than 38 degrees. I am going to measure the dose with a plastic syringe.

3. What are the side effects?
   There are no side effects, but I must not give her too much.

4. I want to make sure that I didn't forget anything. Please, can you explain to me how you are going to give this medicine?
   This medicine is an acetaminophen suspension. It will reduce her temperature when there is a fever. I am going to give her 2 teaspoonfuls or 10 mL every 4 to 6 hours only if she has a fever. I am going to measure the medicine with a plastic syringe.

Very good, I hope that your daughter feels better soon. May all go well.

Thank you very much, Doctor. Goodbye.

1. Because of differences in the use of degrees Centigrade and Fahrenheit in other countries, health care professionals may need to clarify the significance of temperature reading with the patient or parent.

2. Common treatments for fever in the Hispanic culture include the following:
   a. Using ice packs over the head and the abdomen
   b. Giving the patient lots of liquids
   c. Bathing young infants with warm or cool water

3. Patients may refer to their weight using kilograms instead of pounds.

4. The adjective "efectivo(a)" can be used in different contexts in the pharmacy. One can say, "Pague en efectivo," which means "Pay with cash." It also can be used as "La medicina es efectiva," meaning "The medicine is effective."

5. The word "seguro(a)" can be used to say, "La medicina es segura," which means "The medicine is safe (to use)." The phrase "¿Está seguro?" means "Are you sure (certain)?"

Cognados falsos / False cognates

False cognates can lead to misunderstandings between a patient and a pharmacist. Check these out:

- "Últimamente" does not translate as "ultimately." It translates as "lately." For example, "Últimamente he sentido un dolor muy fuerte en la pierna" means "Lately I have felt a strong pain in my leg."
- "Instructions" or "directions" for using a medicine is translated to "instrucciones." When we tell the patient to "follow the directions," we must say "siga las instrucciones." The Spanish word "dirección" refers to someone's street address or cardinal direction (north, south, east, and west). For example, "¿Cuál es su dirección?" is used to say "What is your address?"
- "Molestar" does not translate as sexual molestation. The adjective "molesto" translates to "bothersome" or "nuisance." The verb "molestar" means "to bother or annoy."

Apuntes de gramática / Grammar notes

Present perfect	Example: (haber + past participle) (have + past participle)	He tenido fiebre desde ayer. I have had a fever since yesterday.
Present progressive	Example: (estar + "gerundio") (is + present participle)	Mi hijo está llorando. My son is crying.

Ejercicios / Exercises

I. Haga una pregunta para cada respuesta. (Write a question for each answer.)

1. ¿_____?
   Ella tiene fiebre y llora mucho.

2. ¿_____?
   No estoy seguro pero alrededor de 39°.

3. ¿_____?
   Desde anoche.

4. ¿_____?
   Mucho líquido y jugo, nada más.

II. Escriba los siguientes números y unidades. (Write out the following numbers and units.)
   Ejemplo: 79 kg = setenta y nueve kilogramos.

1. 98.6°F   _____
2. 480 mg / 15 mL   _____
3. 120 mg / 1.2 mL   _____
4. 37.5°C   _____

III. Escriba una oración con las siguientes palabras. (Write a sentence using the following words.)

1. termómetro / oído / calentura

2. agitar / medir / cucharita / niños

3. dar / suspensión / fiebre

IV. Busque en el Internet un sitio en español y escriba un párrafo sobre uno de los siguientes temas.
(Look up an Internet site in Spanish and write a paragraph about one of the following topics.)

1. fiebre

2. termómetro

REFERENCES

1. Takiya L. Fever. In: Berardi RR, Kroon LA, McDermott JH, et al., eds. *Handbook of Nonprescription Drugs.* 15th ed. Washington, DC: American Pharmacists Association; 2006:91–107.
2. Lacy CF, Armstrong LL, Goldman MP, et al. *Drug Information Handbook.* 17th ed. Hudson, Ohio: Lexi-Comp; 2008.
3. Gardner M, Boyce RW, Herrier RN. *Pharmacist–Patient Consultation Program PPCP-Unit I: An Interactive Approach to Verifying Patient Understanding.* New York: Pfizer Educational Services; 1991.

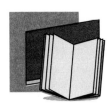

Lección 3 Dolor de cabeza
Lesson 3 Headache

Verbos / Verbs		Presente / Present tense			
		Yo	Él, ella, usted	Mandato	Ejemplos
deprimir(se)	to feel depressed	me deprimo	se deprime	No se deprima*	*El invierno **me deprime**.* *No se deprima por favor.*
enojar(se)	to anger	me enojo	se enoja	No se enoje*	*Por favor, **no se enoje**.* *Ya puedo surtir su receta.*
evitar	to avoid	evito	evita	Evite	***Evite** la luz cuando tenga dolor de cabeza.*
frustrar(se)	to frustrate	(me) frustro	(se) frustra	No se frustre*	***No se frustre**, mejor tome su medicamento.*
fumar	to smoke	fumo	fuma	No fume*	***No fume**; empeora el dolor.*
preocupar(se)	to worry	me preocupo	se preocupa	No se preocupe*	***Me preocupo** por las palpitaciones que siento.*
servir(se)	to serve, to help	me sirve	le sirve	Sirva	*Esta medicina **no le sirve**.*
sufrir	to suffer	sufro	sufre	No sufra*	***Sufro** de migrañas.*

*These commands are frequently used in the negative.

Sustantivos / Nouns

la ansiedad	anxiety
el aura	aura
la bebida	drink
la botella	bottle
el cansancio	fatigue
la comida	food
la cosa	thing
la depresión	depression
la ebriedad, la borrachera (slang)	drunkenness
el enojo	anger
el estrés	stress
el frasco	bottle
la frustración	frustration
la fuerza	force, strength
el insomnio	insomnia
el lado	side
el líquido	liquid
la luz (las luces)	light(s)
la migraña, la jaqueca	migraine
la palpitación	palpitation, throbbing
el pómulo	cheekbone
el refresco	soft drink
la resaca, la cruda (slang)	hangover
el ruido	noise
la tensión	tension
la tristeza	sadness

Adjetivos / Adjectives

alcohólico(a)	alcoholic
borracho(a) (slang)	drunk
brillante	bright
deprimido(a)	depressed
enojado(a)	angry
frustrado(a)	frustrated
fuerte	strong
tenso(a)	tense
triste	sad

Adverbios / Adverbs

abajo	underneath
adentro	inside
afuera	outside
arriba	above
atrás	back
bajo	under
debajo	below
enfrente	in front
a los lados	to the sides
muy	very

Otras expresiones / Other expressions

de vez en cuando	sometimes
desde ayer	since yesterday
desde el mes pasado	since last month
desde la semana pasada	since last week
Lo siento.	I'm sorry.
por ejemplo	for example
¿Qué tan seguido?, ¿Con qué frecuencia?	How often?
¡Qué pena!	How unfortunate!

Preguntas[1]

1. ¿Le duele la cabeza?
2. ¿Dónde le duele? ¿Enfrente, atrás, arriba o a los lados?
3. ¿Cómo es el dolor? ¿Agudo, sordo, fuerte, con palpitaciones?
4. ¿Qué tan seguido tiene dolor de cabeza? ¿Desde cuándo lo ha tenido?
5. ¿Le duelen los pómulos?
6. ¿Ve luces? ¿Tiene aura?
7. ¿Está frustrado(a), tenso(a) o enojado(a)? ¿Siente ansiedad o está bajo mucho estrés?
8. ¿Tiene tristeza o depresión?
9. ¿Qué le calma el dolor?
10. ¿Duerme bien? ¿Tiene insomnio o duerme mucho?
11. ¿Qué le causa el dolor? ¿Qué tipo de comidas o bebidas? ¿Le duele cuando está cansado? ¿El ruido o las luces brillantes le causan dolor?
12. ¿Toma alguna medicina para el dolor? ¿Le sirve?
13. ¿Toma bebidas alcohólicas? ¿Toma café, refrescos, té o chocolate?
14. ¿Fuma?

Recomendaciones

1. Tome esta pastilla. Contiene acetaminofén (250 mg), aspirina (250 mg) y cafeína (65 mg).
2. Si tiene dolor de cabeza, tome de 1 a 2 pastilla(s) cada 4 a 6 horas con comida.

Efectos secundarios (molestias)

Es posible que el medicamento le cause náusea, malestar de estómago o acidez.

Las preguntas fundamentales[2]

1. ¿Para qué es esta medicina?
2. ¿Cómo va a usar esta medicina?
3. ¿Cuáles son los efectos secundarios?
4. Quiero confirmar que no olvidé nada. ¿Ahora, me puede explicar cómo va a usar esta medicina?

Questions

1. Do you have a headache? (Does your head hurt?)
2. Where does it hurt? In front, on the back, on the top, or to the sides?
3. How is the pain? Sharp, dull, strong, (with) throbbing?
4. How often do you have headaches? How long have you had them?
5. Do your cheekbones (sinuses) hurt?
6. Do you see lights? Do you have an aura?
7. Are you frustrated, tense, or angry? Do you feel anxious, or are you under much stress?
8. Do you feel sad or are you depressed? Do you have sadness or depression?
9. What calms the pain?
10. How well do you sleep? Do you have insomnia, or do you sleep a lot?
11. What causes (you) the pain? What type of food or drinks? Does it hurt (you) when you are tired? Does noise or bright lights cause you pain?
12. Do you take some medicine for the pain? Does it help you?
13. Do you drink alcoholic beverages? Do you consume coffee, soft drinks, tea, or chocolate?
14. Do you smoke?

Recommendations

1. Take this pill. It has acetaminophen (250 mg), aspirin (250 mg), and caffeine (65 mg).
2. If you have a headache, take 1 to 2 pills every 4 to 6 hours with food.

Side effects

It is possible that this medication may cause nausea, upset stomach, or heartburn.

Prime questions[2]

1. What is this medication for?
2. How are you going to use this medication?
3. What are the side effects?
4. I want to make sure that I didn't forget anything. Now, can you explain to me how you are going to use this medicine?

Diálogos para el audio

FARMACÉUTICA: Buenos días. Me llamo Thomasa Baker. Soy su farmacéutica. ¿En qué le puedo ayudar?

PACIENTE: *Buenos días, Sra. Baker. Yo me llamo Petra Valdés. Pues mire, últimamente he tenido dolores de cabeza frecuentes y muy fuertes. Ahora tengo un dolor de cabeza muy, muy molesto. ¿Qué me recomienda?*

FARMACÉUTICA: Bueno, tengo que hacerle unas preguntas antes de recomendarle algún producto.

Preguntas[1]

1. ¿Entonces, le duele la cabeza?
   Sí, me duele mucho.

2. ¿Dónde le duele? ¿Enfrente, atrás, arriba o a los lados?
   Me duele la cabeza, en la frente especialmente.

3. ¿Cómo es el dolor? ¿Agudo, sordo, fuerte, con palpitaciones?
   El dolor es sordo y continuo. Pero a veces es agudo con palpitaciones.

4. ¿Qué tan seguido tiene dolor de cabeza? ¿Desde cuándo ha tenido este dolor de cabeza?
   Tengo dolores de cabeza de vez en cuando. He tenido este dolor desde hace 2 días más o menos.

5. ¿Le duelen los pómulos?
   No, no me duelen los pómulos realmente.

6. ¿Ve luces? ¿Tiene aura?
   No, no veo luces, sólo me duele aquí en las sienes arriba de las orejas.

7. ¿Está frustrada, tensa o enojada? ¿Siente ansiedad o está bajo mucho estrés?
   A veces me siento frustrada. ¡No tengo tiempo para descansar! También tengo algo de estrés en el trabajo.

8. ¿Siente tristeza o tiene depresión?
   No, no estoy triste ni tampoco me siento deprimida.

9. ¿Qué le calma el dolor?
   Siento alivio sólo cuando me duermo.

10. ¿Duerme bien? ¿Tiene insomnio o duerme mucho?
    Duermo más o menos bien.

11. ¿Qué le causa el dolor? ¿Qué tipo de comidas o bebidas? ¿Le duele la cabeza cuando está cansada? ¿El ruido o las luces brillantes le causan dolor?
    Creo que el dolor de cabeza es a causa del estrés en el trabajo. Últimamente he trabajado horas extras y también estudio por las noches. No tengo ningún problema con las comidas ni tampoco con los ruidos o las luces.

12. ¿Toma alguna medicina para el dolor? ¿Le sirve?
    Generalmente no tomo nada. La verdad es que no me gusta tomar medicina.

13. ¿Toma bebidas alcohólicas? ¿Toma café, refrescos, té o chocolate?
    Sí, tomo bebidas alcohólicas de vez en cuando pero no soy alcohólica. Tomo café por las mañanas.

14. ¿Fuma?
    No, no fumo.

Recomendaciones

1. Pues, le recomiendo esta medicina. Contiene acetaminofén, aspirina y cafeína.
2. Si tiene dolor de cabeza, tome de 1 a 2 pastillas cada 4 a 6 horas con comida.
3. Si estos dolores de cabeza continúan o empeoran, le recomiendo que consulte a su médico de cabecera.

Efectos secundarios (molestias)

Es posible que el medicamento le cause náusea, malestar de estómago o acidez.

Las preguntas fundamentales[2]

1. ¿Para qué es esta medicina?
   Esta medicina es para aliviar el dolor de cabeza.

2. ¿Cómo va a usar esta medicina?
   Voy a tomar de 1 a 2 pastillas cada 4 a 6 horas, solamente si tengo dolor de cabeza.

3. ¿Cuáles son los efectos secundarios?
   Es posible que la medicina me cause náusea, malestar de estómago o acidez. Por esta razón, debo tomar la medicina con comida siempre.

4. Quiero confirmar que no olvidé nada. ¿Ahora, me puede explicar cómo va a usar esta medicina?
   Sí, claro. Voy a tomar de 1 a 2 pastillas cada 4 a 6 horas, solamente si tengo dolor de cabeza. Debo tomarlas con comida para evitar molestias en el estómago.

◼ *Audio dialogues*

PHARMACIST: Good morning. My name is Thomasa Baker. I am your pharmacist. How can I help you?

PATIENT: *Good morning, Ms. Baker. My name is Petra Valdés. Well, look, lately I have experienced frequent and very painful headaches. Now I have a very bothersome and painful headache. What can you recommend to me?*

PHARMACIST: Well, I need to ask a few questions before I can recommend a product.

Questions[1]

1. So, you have a headache? (Does your head hurt?)
   Yes, my head hurts a lot.

2. Where does it hurt? In front, on the back, on top, or to the sides?
   My forehead hurts especially.

3. How is the pain? Sharp, dull, strong, throbbing?
   The pain is dull and constant. But at times the pain is sharp and throbbing.

4. How often do you have headaches? How long have you had them?
   I have headaches every now and then. I have had this headache since 2 days ago, more or less.

5. Do your cheekbones (sinuses) hurt?
   No, my cheekbones don't really hurt.

6. Do you see lights? Do you have an aura?
   No, I do not see lights. It just hurts here, in my temples, above my ears.

7. Are you frustrated, tense, or angry? Do you feel anxious or are you under much stress?
   Sometimes I feel frustrated. I do not have time to rest! I also have some stress at work.

8. Do you feel sad or feel depressed?
   No, I do not feel sad, nor do I feel depressed.

9. What calms the pain?
   I feel better when I sleep—if I am successful in sleeping.

10. How well do you sleep? Do you have insomnia, or do you sleep a lot?
    I sleep more or less well.

11. What causes (you) the pain? What type of food or drinks? Do you have pain when you are tired? Do noise or bright lights cause you pain?
    I think that the headaches are caused by the stress at work. Lately, I have worked extra hours, and I also go to school at night. I don't have any problems with food, noise, or lights.

12. Do you take some medicine for the pain? Does it help you?
    Generally, I do not take anything. The truth is that I do not like to take medicine.

13. Do you drink alcoholic beverages? Do you consume coffee, soft drinks, tea, or chocolate?
    Yes, I drink alcohol once in a while, but I am not an alcoholic. I drink a cup of coffee in the mornings.

14. Do you smoke?
    No, I do not smoke.

Recommendations

1. Well, I recommend this medication. It contains acetaminophen, aspirin, and caffeine.
2. If you have a headache, take 1 to 2 pills every 4 to 6 hours with food.
3. If these headaches continue or should become worse, I recommend that you consult with your primary care physician.

Side effects

It is possible that this medication may cause nausea, upset stomach, or heartburn.

Prime questions[2]

1. What is this medication for?
   This medicine is for relieving my headache.

2. How are you going to use this medication?
   I will take 1 to 2 pills every 4 to 6 hours only if I have a headache.

3. What are the side effects?
   It is possible that this medication may cause me nausea, upset stomach, or heartburn. For this reason, I should always take this medicine with food.

4. I want to make sure that I didn't forget anything. Now, can you explain to me how you are going to use this medicine?
   Yes, of course. I am going to take 1 to 2 pills every 4 to 6 hours only if I have a headache. I should take them with food to avoid an upset stomach.

in the Hispanic culture include the following:
o" or other soups
on
in women)
e the pain

otes

ast participle)   Ella <u>está deprimida</u>.
ple)   She <u>is depressed</u>.

ciple)   Ella <u>se siente deprimida</u>.
ciple)   She <u>feels depressed</u>.

Ejercicios / *Exercises*

I. Haga una pregunta para cada respuesta. (Write a question for each answer.)

1. ¿_____?

   Sí, si tomo bebidas alcohólicas me da cruda.

2. ¿_____?

   Me dan muchas palpitaciones [en las sienes] cuando me duele la cabeza.

3. ¿_____?

   Si tengo migraña veo luces y un aura alrededor de las cosas.

4. ¿_____?

   Me lo causan la tensión, el cansancio y la frustración.

II. Escoja el antónimo correcto. (Select the correct antonym.)

_____1. abajo   a. adentro
_____2. enfrente   b. arriba
_____3. insomnio   c. alegría
_____4. afuera   d. atrás
_____5. tristeza   e. sueño

III. Escriba una oración o pregunta con las siguientes palabras. (Write a sentence or question with the following words.)

1. evitar / bebidas

2. doler(se) / arriba

3. estar / enojar

4. servir / cruda

IV. Busque en el Internet un sitio en español y escriba un párrafo sobre uno de los siguientes temas.
(Look up an Internet site in Spanish and write a paragraph about one of the following topics.)

1. migrañas

2. dependencia a las drogas, al tabaco o al alcohol

V. Gramática / Grammar
Relacione el adjetivo con su sustantivo. Llene los espacios con el adjetivo o el sustantivo apropiado.
(Match the adjective [past participle] with its noun. Fill in the blanks with the appropriate adjective or noun.)

   Ejemplo: ¿Tiene tensión? Sí, estoy tensa.

1. ¿Está _____? Sí, tengo frustración.
2. ¿Tiene _____? No, no me siento triste.
3. ¿Se siente deprimida? Sí, tengo_____.
4. ¿Están _____? Sí, tenemos cansancio.
5. ¿Está enojada? No, no tengo _____.

REFERENCES

1. Remington TL. Headache. In: Berardi RR, Kroon LA, McDermott JH, et al., eds. *Handbook of Nonprescription Drugs.* 15th ed. Washington, DC: American Pharmacists Association; 2006:69–90.
2. Gardner M, Boyce RW, Herrier RN. *Pharmacist–Patient Consultation Program PPCP-Unit I: An Interactive Approach to Verifying Patient Understanding.* New York: Pfizer Educational Services; 1991.

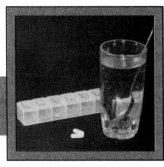

Acidez y reflujo
Heartburn and reflux

Verbos / Verbs		Presente / Present tense			
		Yo	Él, ella, usted	Mandato	Ejemplos
acostar(se)	to go to bed	me acuesto	se acuesta	Acuéstese	*No **se acueste** después de comer.*
agachar(se)	to bend over	me agacho	se agacha	Agáchese	*Me duele el estómago cuando **me agacho.***
apretar	to squeeze, to press	aprieto	aprieta	Apriete	*No use ropa que **le apriete.***
ayudar	to help	ayudo	ayuda	Ayude	***Ayúdeme** por favor.*
bajar de peso	to lose weight	bajo de peso	baja	Baje	***Baje** de peso para mejorar su salud.*
disolver	to dissolve	disuelvo	disuelve	Disuelva	***Disuelva** la tableta en agua.*
empezar	to begin	empiezo	empieza	Empiece	***Empiece** la medicina hoy mismo.*
eructar	to burp	eructo	eructa	Eructe	*¿**Eructa** mucho después de comer?*
explicar	to explain	explico	explica	Explíqueme (*Explain to me*)	***Explíqueme** dónde tiene el dolor exactamente.*
extender	to extend	extiendo	extiende	Extienda	*El dolor se me **extiende** al pecho.*
masticar	to chew	mastico	mastica	Mastique	***Mastique** la pastilla, no la trague.*
neutralizar	to neutralize	neutralizo	neutraliza	Neutralice	*Esta medicina **neutraliza** el ácido estomacal.*
pasar	to pass through (e.g., stomach)	lo paso	lo pasa	Páselo	*La medicina **pasa** de la boca al esófago.*
preferir	to prefer	prefiero	prefiere	Prefiera	***Prefiero** tomar pastillas, no jarabes.*
prevenir	to prevent	prevengo	previene	Prevenga	*Este medicamento **previene** el exceso de ácido en el estómago.*
producir	to produce	produzco	produce	Produzca	*La medicina no **produce** efectos secundarios.*

continued on p. 38

Verbos / Verbs		Presente / Present tense			
		Yo	Él, ella, usted	Mandato	Ejemplos
provocar	to provoke	provoco	me provoca, le provoca	Provoque	*Esta medicina* **me provoca** *náuseas.*
repetir	to belch, to repeat	repito	repite	Repita (*Repeat*)	*Esta pastilla evita que* **repita** *demasiado.* **Repita** *la dosis en la tarde.*
toser	to cough	toso	tose	Tosa	*Con la acidez,* **toso** *mucho.*
tragar	to swallow	trago	traga	Trague	*No* **trague** *la pastilla, mastíquela.*
tratar	to treat (medical), to try	trato	trata	Trate	**Trate** *los síntomas de acidez con antiácidos.*

El sistema digestivo (parte alta) / Digestive system (upper portion)

la boca	mouth
los dientes	teeth
la epiglotis	epiglottis
el esófago	esophagus
el estómago	stomach
la garganta	throat
la lengua	tongue
las papilas gustativas	taste buds
el pecho	chest
el vientre	abdomen

Sustantivos / Nouns

la acidez	acidity, heartburn
el ácido cítrico	citric acid
las agruras*	acidity
el ajo	garlic
el aluminio	aluminum
el antiácido	antacid
el antihistamínico	antihistamine
el asco*	nausea
el bicarbonato de sodio	sodium bicarbonate
la cafeína	caffeine
el calcio	calcium
la cebolla	onion
la diarrea	diarrhea
la distensión abdominal	abdominal distension
la esofaguitis	esophagitis
la experiencia	experience
la grasa	fat
el hábito	habit
el hierro	iron
el hipo	hiccups
la incomodidad	discomfort
la indigestión	indigestion
la inflamación	inflammation
la inflamación abdominal	bloating
el malestar	discomfort
el mareo	dizziness, nausea
la menta	mint
la(s) porción(es)	portion(s)
el reflujo	reflux
la ropa	clothes
la sal	salt
la sangre	blood
el (los) signo(s)	sign(s)
el (los) síntoma(s)	symptom(s)
el sueño	sleep, dream
la tableta	tablet
la taza	cup
la úlcera	ulcer
el vómito	vomit

Adjetivos / Adjectives

ácido(a)	acid
agrio(a)	sour, acid, tart
amargo(a)	bitter
apretado(a)	tight-fitting
condimentado(a)	spicy, seasoned
efervescente	effervescent
esofágico(a)	esophageal
mareado(a)	dizzy, seasick
pequeño(a)	small
picante	hot, spicy

Otras expresiones / Other expressions

después (de)	after
durante	during
Hágalo.	Do it.
inmediatamente	immediately
luego	later
Permítame.	Allow me.
pronto	sooner
Tengo ganas de vomitar.	I feel like vomiting.

---

*Nontechnical term that may be popular in certain Spanish-speaking populations.

Preguntas[1]

1. ¿Le duele el estómago? ¿Tiene malestar en el pecho?
2. Describa cómo se siente. ¿Eructa con frecuencia? ¿Tiene náusea, inflamación abdominal o indigestión? ¿Tiene ganas de vomitar? ¿Tiene tos?
3. ¿Le duele o le arde? ¿El dolor se le extiende (se le va) al pecho, a la espalda o a la garganta?
4. ¿A qué hora del día siente incomodidad? ¿Le duele el estómago o la garganta después de comer? ¿Le duele más cuando se acuesta? ¿Cuando se agacha?
5. ¿A qué hora come durante el día? ¿Se siente peor con ciertas comidas o bebidas?
6. ¿Qué le calma el dolor? ¿Hay algún medicamento que le ayude?
7. ¿Tiene molestias cuando traga? ¿Tiene sangre en la garganta o en la boca? (Si es así, refiéralo al doctor.)
8. ¿Fuma?

Recomendaciones

I. Antiácidos: Úselos para tratar los síntomas de acidez.
Este antiácido contiene calcio de 500 (quinientos) mg.
Los antiácidos pueden calmarle el malestar estomacal.

1. Mastique de 1 a 2 tabletas de cuatro a seis veces al día cuando sea necesario.
2. Tómelo inmediatamente después de las comidas o antes de acostarse si es necesario.
3. No lo tome por más de 2 semanas. Si lo necesita por más tiempo, consulte a su doctor.

Otras recomendaciónes:
1. No lo tome con productos de hierro.
2. Dígame si empieza a tomar otras medicinas.
3. Si toma una suspensión, agítela bien antes de tomarla.
Si prefiere, tome un antiácido efervescente. Contiene bicarbonato de sodio, ácido cítrico y aspirina.

Para tomarlo
1. Disuelva 1 a 2 tabletas en una taza pequeña (de 4 a 6 onzas) de agua y tómelas.
2. Hágalo cuando tenga agruras o acidez.
No puede darle este medicamento a los niños porque contiene aspirina.

Efectos secundarios (molestias)
Los medicamentos de magnesio pueden causarle diarrea.
Los medicamentos de calcio y aluminio pueden causarle estreñimiento.

II. Los antihistamínicos para el estómago.* Úselos para prevenir el reflujo.
Esta medicina se llama ranitidina de 75 mg (setenta y cinco).
Le ayuda a su estómago a no producir demasiado ácido.
Tome 1 tableta de 30 a 60 minutos antes de una comida que le provoque acidez.

Efectos secundarios (molestias)
El medicamento puede provocarle dolor de cabeza, mareo o sueño.

Cambios en el estilo de vida
Es necesario que cambie algunos hábitos para mejorar su digestión.
1. Coma porciones más pequeñas.
2. No se acueste en las siguientes 3 horas después de comer.
3. Evite comidas como el chocolate, la comida grasosa, ajo, cebollas, mentas o comida picante o condimentada.
4. Evite fumar y también la cafeína y el alcohol.
5. Evite tomar aspirina o ibuprofeno.
6. No use ropa apretada.
7. Baje de peso.

Las preguntas fundamentales[2]
1. ¿Para qué es esta medicina?
2. ¿Cómo va a tomar esta medicina?
3. ¿Cuáles son los efectos secundarios?
4. Quiero confirmar si no olvidé algo. ¿Ahora, me puede explicar cómo va a tomar esta medicina?

---

*These antihistamines may be used at nonprescription dose (half) for preventing heartburn.

Questions[1]

1. Does your stomach hurt? Do you have discomfort in your chest?
2. Describe how you feel. Do you burp often? Do you have nausea, bloating, or indigestion? Do you feel like vomiting? Do you have a cough?
3. Does it hurt or burn? Does it extend (go) to the chest, back, or throat?
4. At what times during the day do you feel discomfort? Does your stomach or throat hurt after eating? Does it hurt when you lie down? When you bend over?
5. When do you eat during the day? Do you feel worse with certain foods or drinks?
6. What relieves the pain? Is there a medication that helps you?
7. Does it bother you when you swallow? Have you had any blood in your throat or mouth? (If so, refer to the doctor.)
8. Do you smoke?

Recommendations

I. Antacids: Use them to treat heartburn symptoms.

This antacid has calcium of 500 mg.

Antacids can relieve an upset stomach.

1. Chew 1 to 2 tablets four to six times a day as needed.
2. Take immediately after meals or at bedtime as needed.
3. Do not take for more than 2 weeks. If you need to take it for a longer time, consult your doctor.

Other recommendations:

1. Do not take with iron products.
2. Tell me if you begin to take any new medication.
3. If you are taking a suspension, shake it well before using.

If you prefer, take an effervescent antacid. It contains sodium bicarbonate, citric acid, and aspirin.

To take it

1. Dissolve 1 to 2 tablets in a small glass (4–6 ounces) of water, and drink it.
2. Do this when you have acidity or heartburn.

Do not give this medication to children, because it contains aspirin.

Side effects

Magnesium products can cause diarrhea.

Calcium and aluminum products can cause constipation.

II. Antihistamines for the stomach. Use them to prevent reflux.

This medicine is called ranitidine 75 mg.

It helps your stomach not to produce too much acid.

Take 1 tablet 30 to 60 minutes before a meal that causes heartburn.

Side effects

The medication can cause headache, dizziness, or drowsiness.

Lifestyle changes

It is necessary to change some habits to improve your digestion.

1. Eat smaller meals (portions).
2. Do not lie down for 3 hours after eating.
3. Avoid foods such as chocolate, fatty foods, garlic, onions, mints, or spicy foods.
4. Avoid smoking and also caffeine and alcohol.
5. Avoid taking aspirin or ibuprofen.
6. Do not wear tight-fitting clothes.
7. Lose weight.

Prime questions[2]

1. What is this medication for?
2. How are you going to use this medication?
3. What are the side effects?
4. I want to confirm that I didn't forget something. Now, can you explain to me how you are going to take this medicine?

Diálogos para el audio

FARMACÉUTICA: Buenos días. Soy la Dra. Martínez. ¿En qué le puedo servir?

PACIENTE: *Buenos días, doctora. Soy Manuel Bejarano. Pues, he tenido algunos problemas en el estómago y el pecho. El doctor me dio esta receta, pero ¿me puede recomendar algo más?*

FARMACÉUTICA: Claro que sí. Pero primero necesito hacerle algunas preguntas.

PACIENTE: *Por supuesto, doctora.*

Preguntas[1]

1. ¿Le duele el estómago? ¿Tiene malestar en el pecho?
   Sí, me duele el estómago y tengo malestar en el pecho, pero no muy fuerte.

2. Describa cómo se siente. ¿Eructa con frecuencia? ¿Tiene náusea, inflamación abdominal o indigestión? ¿Tiene tos?
   Sí, eructo mucho, tengo indigestión y siento el vientre inflamado. Pero no tengo ganas de vomitar. Y no tengo tos.

3. ¿Le duele o le arde? ¿El dolor se le extiende al pecho, a la espalda o a la garganta?
   No me arde tanto el estómago, ni se me va a otras partes del cuerpo.

4. ¿A qué hora del día siente incomodidad? ¿Le duele el estómago o la garganta después de comer? ¿Le duele más cuando se acuesta? ¿Cuando se agacha?
   Me duele el estómago después de comer, cuando me acuesto y a veces cuando me agacho.

5. ¿A qué hora come durante el día? ¿Se siente peor con ciertas comidas o bebidas?
   No como hasta en la noche porque trabajo todo el día. Entonces, estoy comiendo después de las 7:00 de la tarde. Con la comida picante o el café me siento peor.

6. ¿Qué le calma el dolor? ¿Hay algún medicamento que le ayude?
   Ahora, nada me calma el dolor y no he tomado ningún medicamento.

7. ¿Tiene molestias cuando traga? ¿Tiene sangre en la garganta o en la boca?
   No, no tengo molestias cuando trago ni tengo sangre en la boca ni en la garganta.

8. ¿Fuma?
   Sí, fumo durante los fines de semana.

Recomendación 1

Voy a recomendarle un medicamento para la acidez. El doctor ya le dio una receta para el reflujo. Pero, tiene que volver con su doctor si los síntomas continúan por más de 2 semanas.

Este antiácido contiene calcio de 500 (quinientos) mg y es para la acidez. Los antiácidos pueden calmarle el malestar estomacal.
1. Mastique de 1 a 2 tabletas de cuatro a seis veces al día cuando sea necesario.
2. Tómelo después de las comidas o antes de acostarse cuando sea necesario.

Si prefiere, tome un antiácido efervescente. Contiene bicarbonato de sodio, ácido cítrico y aspirina.

Para tomarlo
1. Disuelva 1 a 2 tabletas en una taza pequeña (de 4 a 6 onzas) de agua y tómelas.
2. Hágalo cuando tenga agruras o acidez.

No puede darle este medicamento a los niños porque contiene aspirina.

Efectos secundarios (molestias)

El calcio le puede causar estreñimiento.

Recomendación 2

La medicina que su doctor le recetó para el reflujo es un antihistamínico. Esta medicina se llama ranitidina es de 75 mg. Le ayuda a su estómago a no producir demasiado ácido. Tome 1 tableta de 30 a 60 minutos antes de una comida que le provoque acidez.

Efectos secundarios (molestias)

El medicamento puede provocarle dolor de cabeza, mareo o sueño.

Cambios en el estilo de vida

Le voy a hacer unas sugerencias para que cambie algunas cosas en su estilo de vida.

Es necesario que cambie algunos hábitos para mejorar su digestión.
1. Coma porciones más pequeñas.
2. No se acueste en las siguientes 3 horas después de comer.
3. Evite la comida picante o condimentada. También es mejor evitar el chocolate, la comida grasosa, ajo, cebolla y mentas.
4. Evite fumar y también la cafeína y el alcohol. Me gustaría hablar con usted otro día para ayudarle a dejar de fumar.

También es bueno que
1. Evite tomar aspirina o ibuprofeno.
2. No use ropa apretada.
3. Baje de peso.

Las preguntas fundamentales[2]

1. ¿Para qué son estas medicinas?
   Son para la acidez y el reflujo.

2. ¿Cómo va a tomar estas medicinas?
   Del antiácido de calcio, voy a masticar de 1 a 2 tabletas de cuatro a seis veces al día, cuando sea necesario para la acidez o me puedo tomar un antiácido efervescente.
   De la ranitidina, voy a tomar una tableta antes de las comidas fuentes para prevenir el reflujo.

3. ¿Cuáles son las molestias?
   El calcio me puede causar estreñimiento. Y la ranitidina me puede causar dolor de cabeza, mareo o sueño.

4. Quiero confirmar si no olvidé algo. Ahora, ¿me puede explicar cómo va a tomar estas medicinas?
   Voy a masticar el antiácido 1 a 2 tabletas de cuatro a seis veces al día si es necesario para la acidez. Para el reflujo, voy a tomarla antes de comer. Debo evitar la comida picante y el café.

Muy bien, Señor Bejarano. Que se sienta mejor.

Muchas gracias por su ayuda, doctora.

◼ *Audio dialogues*

PHARMACIST: Good morning, I am Dr. Martínez. How can I help you?

PATIENT: *Good morning, Doctor. I am Manuel Bejarano. Well, I have had some problems in my stomach and in my chest. My doctor gave me this prescription, but can you recommend something else for me?*

PHARMACIST: Of course. But first I need to ask you a few questions.

PATIENT: *Of course, Doctor.*

Questions[1]

1. Does your stomach hurt? Do you have discomfort in your chest?
   Yes, my stomach hurts and I have chest discomfort, but not very strong.

2. Describe how you feel. Do you burp often? Do you have nausea, bloating, or indigestion? Do you have a cough?
   Yes, I burp a lot, I have indigestion, and I feel my abdomen is swollen. But I do not feel like vomiting. And I don't cough.

3. Does it hurt or burn? Does it extend to the chest, back, or throat?
   My stomach doesn't burn that much. Nor does it go to other parts of my body.

4. At what times during the day do you feel discomfort? Does your stomach or throat hurt after you eat? Does it hurt when you lie down? When you bend over?
   My stomach hurts after eating, when I lie down, and sometimes when I bend over.

5. When do you eat during the day? Do you feel worse with certain foods or drinks?
   I don't eat until the evening because I work all day. So I am eating after 7:00 in the evening. When I eat certain spicy foods or coffee, I feel worse.

6. What relieves the pain? Is there a medication that helps you?
   Now, nothing relieves the pain. I haven't taken any medications.

7. Does it bother you when you swallow? Have you had any blood in your throat or mouth?
   No, I don't have any discomfort when I swallow, nor do I have blood in my mouth.

8. Do you smoke?
   Yes, I smoke during the weekends.

Recommendation 1

I am going to recommend a medication for heartburn for you. Your doctor already gave you a prescription for reflux (gastroesophageal reflux disease). But you have to return to your doctor if the symptoms continue for more than 2 weeks.

This antacid contains calcium 500 mg and is for heartburn. Antacids can relieve an upset stomach.
1. Chew 1 to 2 tablets four to six times a day as needed.
2. Take after meals and at bedtime as needed.

If you prefer, take an effervescent antacid. It contains sodium bicarbonate, citric acid, and aspirin.

To take it
1. Dissolve 1 to 2 tablets in a small glass (4–6 ounces) of water, and drink it.
2. Do this when you have acidity or heartburn.
Do not give this medication to children, because it contains aspirin.

Side effects

Calcium can cause constipation.

Recommendation 2

The medicine that your doctor prescribed for you for reflux is an antihistamine. This medicine is called ranitidine 75 mg. It helps your stomach not produce too much acid.
Take 1 tablet 30 to 60 minutes before a meal that causes heartburn.

Side effects

The medication can cause headache, dizziness, or drowsiness.

Lifestyle changes

I am going to make a few suggestions so that you can make some lifestyle changes.
It is necessary that you change some habits to improve your digestion.
1. Eat smaller meals (portions).
2. Do not lie down for 3 hours after eating.
3. Avoid spicy or seasoned foods. Also, it is better to avoid chocolate, fatty foods, garlic, onions, and mints.
4. Avoid smoking and also caffeine and alcohol. I would like to talk with you another day about quitting smoking.

It is also good if you
1. Avoid taking aspirin or ibuprofen.
2. Do not wear tight-fitting clothes.
3. Lose weight.

Prime questions[2]

1. What are these medications for?
   They are for heartburn and reflux.

2. How are you going to take these medications?
   With the calcium antacid, I am going to chew 1 to 2 tablets 4 to 6 times a day when it is necessary for heartburn, or I can take an effervescent antacid.
   With the ranitidine, I am going to take a tablet before heavy meals.

3. What are the side effects?
   The calcium can cause me constipation. And the ranitidine can cause me headaches, dizziness, or drowsiness.

4. I want to confirm that I didn't forget something. Now, can you explain to me how you are going to take these medicines?
   I am going to chew 1 to 2 antacid tablets four to six times a day if it is necessary for heartburn. For the reflux, I am going to take it before eating. I should avoid spicy foods and coffee.

Very well, Mr. Bejarano. May you feel better.

Thank you very much for your help, Doctor.

De la cultura / About the culture

1. The noun "mareo" ("dizziness") should not be confused with "marea" ("ocean tide"). Interestingly, the adjective "mareado(a)" means "dizzy" or "seasick."

2. Milk products or "productos lácteos" (e.g., yogurt) are often taken for mild stomach discomforts.

3. Some technical terms may not be familiar to patients. Examples of technical or formal Spanish words include "reflujo," "acidez," and "distensión abdominal." Therefore, it is important to be able to describe some terms in simple Spanish so that the patient can understand better.

4. In the English language, health care professionals frequently ask, "Do you experience [nausea]?" This can be translated literally and awkwardly to "¿Experimenta [náusea]?" However, in Spanish it is more common to use the verb *to have* ("tener"). For example, "¿Tiene [náusea]?" or "Do you have [nausea]?"

5. When "luego" is doubled as "luego luego" it does not mean "later," but rather "immediately." For example, "Necesito la medicina luego luego" would mean "I need the medicine immediately."

Apuntes de gramática / Grammar notes

Stem-changing verbs

Example: repetir (to repeat) → repite (he or she repeats or you [formal] repeat)

prevenir (to prevent) → previene (he or she prevents or you [formal] prevent)

acostarse (to lie down) → me acuesto (I lie down)

Verb following preposition

In Spanish, after a preposition, always use the infinitive of the verb.

Example: después de comer (after eating)

para disolver (to dissolve)

Ejercicios / Exercises

I. Llene los espacios en blanco con la palabra apropiada o el verbo conjugado. (Fill in the blanks with the appropriate word or conjugated verb.)

1. (acostarse) ___ _____ cuando (sentir) _____ un malestar en el estómago.

2. (empezar, tener) _____ a _____ los síntomas de _____ y

   _____ cuando tengo acidez.

3. Evite comidas como _____, _____ y _____ para (prevenir)

   _____ reflujo.

II. Use un sinónimo o describa los siguientes términos con sus propias palabras. (Use a synonym or describe the following terms with your own words.)

1. indigestión: _____

2. náusea: _____

3. ácido: _____

4. acidez: _____

5. efervescente: _____

6. distensión abdominal: _____

7. reflujo: _____

III. Escriba un antónimo para las siguientes palabras. (Write an antonym for the following words.)

1. después _____

2. luego _____

3. inmediatamente _____

IV. Haga una pregunta para cada respuesta. (Write a question for each answer.)

1. ¿_____?
   Tengo dolor de estómago.

2. ¿_____?
   Es ardor. A veces se me extiende al pecho y a la garganta.

3. ¿_____?
   Me dan acedías después de comer.

4. ¿_____?
   Es peor cuando me agacho pero no cuando me acuesto.

5. ¿_____?
   Sí, después de tomar café o cuando como con picante.

V. Escriba una oración con las siguientes palabras usando distintos tiempos verbales. (Write a sentence with the following words using different verb tenses.)

1. necesito / comida / eructar

2. tener / agruras / antiácidos

3. disolver / tableta / agua

4. antiácido / contener / aluminio

5. evitar / grasa / comida

6. prevenir / acidez / dieta

VI. Escriba las siguientes oraciones en otras palabras. (Write the following sentences using different words.)

Ejemplo: ¿Ha tenido reflujo? ¿Le causa incomodidad?
En otras palabras: ¿Tiene reflujo? ¿Le molesta mucho?

1. Tengo dolor de estómago. _____

2. Toso durante toda la noche. _____

3. Ha disuelto la medicina. _____

4. ¿Le sirve el antiácido? _____

VII. Conteste las siguientes preguntas en español. (Answer the following questions in Spanish.)

1. ¿Cuáles son otros contenidos de los antiácidos?

2. ¿Diga algunas presentaciones de los antiácidos?

3. Describa cómo pasa la comida a través del sistema digestivo.

VIII. Busque en el Internet un sitio en español sobre uno de los temas siguientes. Escriba un párrafo sencillo para explicarle a un paciente. (Look up an Internet site in Spanish about one of the following topics. Write a simple paragraph to explain it to a patient.)

1. antiácidos

2. antihistamínico (para el estómago)

3. acidez

4. reflujo

5. úlcera

REFERENCES

1. Zweber A, Berardi RR. Heartburn and dyspepsia. In: Berardi RR, Kroon LA, McDermott JH, et al., eds. *Handbook of Nonprescription Drugs.* 15th ed. Washington, DC: American Pharmacists Association; 2006:265–82.
2. Gardner M, Boyce RW, Herrier RN. *Pharmacist–Patient Consultation Program PPCP-Unit I: An Interactive Approach to Verifying Patient Understanding.* New York: Pfizer Educational Services; 1991.

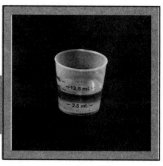

Capítulo / Chapter 3

Tos, resfrío, alergias
Cough, cold, allergies

Verbos / Verbs		Presente / Present tense			
		Yo	Él, ella, usted	Mandato	Ejemplos
beber	to drink	bebo	bebe	Beba	*Beba más líquidos para ayudarle con la tos.*
chupar	to retain in the mouth until it dissolves, to suck on	chupo	chupa	Chupe	*No mastique la pastilla, chúpela.*
consultar	to consult	consulto	consulta	Consulte	*Si la tos empeora, consulte a su médico.*
contagiar(se)	to contaminate (person to person)	contagio	contagia	No contagie	*No le estornude en la cara, lo puede contagiar.*
cubrir(se)	to cover	(me) cubro	(se) cubre	Cúbrase	*Cúbrase la boca para toser.*
curar	to cure	curo	cura	Cure	*El medicamento no cura el resfrío pero sí alivia los síntomas.*
escoger	to choose	escojo	escoge	Escoja	*Los niños escogen el sabor a uva en el jarabe para la tos.*
estornudar	to sneeze	estornudo	estornuda	Estornude	*Cuando estornude por favor cúbrase la boca con un Kleenex.*
fluir	to flow	fluyo	fluye	—	*El catarro me fluye como agua.*
lavar(se)	to wash with soap	(me) lavo	(se) lava	Lávese	*Lávese las manos.*
manejar	to drive	manejo	maneja	Maneje	*No maneje después de tomar el medicamento.*
quitar	to get rid of	quito	quita	Quite	*No se me quita la tos.*
utilizar	to utilize	utilizo	utiliza	Utilice	*Utilice la jeringa de plástico para medir el elixir.*
vomitar	to vomit	vomito	vomita	Vomite	*¿Tiene ganas de vomitar?*

Las partes del sistema respiratorio / Parts of the respiratory system

los bronquios	bronchi
las fosas, las ventanas nasales	nostrils
la garganta	throat
la laringe	larynx
la nariz	nose
el (los) pómulo(s)	cheekbone(s)
el (los) pulmón(es)	lung(s)
los senos nasales	nasal sinuses
la tráquea	trachea

Sustantivos / Nouns

la advertencia	warning
la cantidad	quantity
el catarro	runny nose
la comezón	itchiness
la confusión	confusion
la congestión del pecho	chest congestion
la consistencia	consistency
los escalofríos	chills
el estornudo	sneeze
el expectorante	expectorant
la flema	phlegm
las gárgaras	gargles
el insomnio	insomnia
la irritabilidad	irritability
la irritación	irritation
la mucosa	mucus
la nariz tapada	congested nose
el nerviosismo	nervousness
la picazón	itchiness (stronger)
la somnolencia	drowsiness (medicine or disease)
el sueño	sleepiness (natural cause), dream
la tos	cough
el trocisco	troche
el vómito	vomit

Adjetivos / Adjectives

amarillento(a)	yellowish
claro(a)	clear
confuso(a)	confusing
enrojecido(a)	reddened
espeso(a)	thick
expectorante	expectorant
flojo(a)	loose (cough)
irritable	irritable
lloroso(a)	tearful, weeping
nervioso(a)	nervous
profundo(a)	deep
rojo(a)	red
seco(a)	dry
terco(a)	stubborn
transparente	transparent
verdoso(a)	greenish

Otras expresiones / Other expressions

las bolsas debajo de los ojos	bags under the eyes
estar congestionado	to be congested
haga gárgaras	gargle [command]
mientras	while
poco(a)	a little
tener flema	to have phlegm
Tengo algo de . . .	I have a slight (somewhat of) . . .

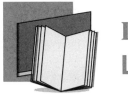

Lección 1 Tos
Lesson 1 Cough

Preguntas[1]

1. ¿Desde cuándo tiene tos?
2. ¿Cómo es la tos? ¿Es seca o tiene flema?
3. Describa la flema.
   – ¿Qué consistencia tiene? ¿Es espesa o líquida? ¿Fluye fácilmente?
   – ¿De qué color es? ¿Contiene sangre? ¿Es transparente, amarillenta o verdosa?
   – ¿Cuánta flema tiene? ¿Mucha o poca?
4. ¿Le duele el pecho cuando tose?
5. ¿Fuma?
6. ¿Tiene otros síntomas?
7. ¿Qué medicamentos toma para la tos?

Recomendación

Este medicamento puede aliviar los síntomas pero no cura la enfermedad.

Guaifenesin 100 mg y dextromethorphan 10 mg por cada 5 ml (1 cucharadita)

Esta medicina contiene dos medicamentos.
Uno es guaifenesin, un expectorante que le ayuda a hacer la flema más líquida y clara.
El otro es dextromethorphan, que le ayuda a controlar la tos.

Adultos: Tome de 1 a 2 cucharaditas de este jarabe cada 4 horas cuando sea necesario para aliviar la tos.

Efectos secundarios (molestias)

Le puede causar somnolencia, nerviosismo, irritabilidad o confusión.

Otras recomendaciones

1. No maneje mientras esté tomando esta medicina.
2. Beba mucha agua.

Las preguntas fundamentales[2]

1. ¿Para qué es esta medicina?
2. ¿Cómo va a usar esta medicina?
3. ¿Cuáles son los efectos secundarios?
4. Me gustaría ver si le expliqué bien. Por favor, dígame cómo va a usar esta medicina.

Questions[1]

1. How long have you had a cough?
2. How is the cough? Is it dry or do you have phlegm?
3. Describe the phlegm.
    – What is the consistency? Is it thick or thin? Does it flow easily?
    – What color? Does it have blood? Is it transparent, yellowish, or greenish?
    – How much phlegm do you have? Is there a lot or a little?
4. Does your chest hurt when you cough?
5. Do you smoke?
6. Do you have other symptoms?
7. What medications do you take for the cough?

Recommendation

This medication can alleviate the symptoms but not cure the illness.

Guaifenesin 100 mg and dextromethorphan 10 mg in each 5 ml (1 teaspoonful)

This medicine contains two medications.
One is guaifenesin, an expectorant that helps make the phlegm more liquid and clear.
The other is dextromethorphan, which helps control (suppress) the cough.

Adults: Take 1 to 2 teaspoons of this syrup every 4 hours as needed to alleviate the cough.

Side effects

It can cause drowsiness, nervousness, irritability, or confusion.

Other recommendations

1. Do not drive while taking this medication.
2. Drink lots of water.

Prime questions[2]

1. What is this medication for?
2. How are you going to use this medication?
3. What are the side effects?
4. I would like to see if I explained it well to you. Please tell me how you are going to use this medicine.

Diálogos para el audio

FARMACÉUTICA: Buenos días. Soy la Sra. Chang-Uriarte. Soy la farmacéutica. Dígame, ¿cómo la puedo ayudar? ¿Cómo se siente?

PACIENTE: *Buenos días, Sra. Chang. Me llamo Dorotea Huerta. Pues, sabe que ando con una tos muy terca. No se me quita con nada ni siquiera con té de orégano ni el de limón. En las noches, toso más; no dejo dormir a nadie. ¿Qué me recomienda tomar?*

Preguntas[1]

1. ¿Desde cuándo tiene tos?
   He tenido esta tos desde el fin de semana pasado.

2. ¿Cómo es la tos? ¿Es seca o tiene flema?
   Es tos con flema.

3. Describa la flema.
   Pues, es flema.

   Lo que quiero decir es . . . ¿qué consistencia tiene? ¿Es espesa o líquida? ¿Fluye fácilmente?
   Es líquida.

   ¿De qué color es? ¿Contiene sangre? ¿Es transparente, amarillenta o verdosa?
   No, no tiene sangre. Es clara.

   ¿Cuánta flema tiene? ¿Mucha o poca?
   Tengo algo de flema.

4. ¿Le duele el pecho cuando tose?
   No, no me duele el pecho realmente, pero ya estoy cansada de toser porque no me deja dormir.

5. ¿Fuma?
   No, no fumo.

6. ¿Tiene otros síntomas?
   No, no creo. Hace un par de semanas tuve un resfriado muy fuerte que me contagió mi marido. Pero no guardé cama. Seguí trabajando en la tienda mi horario normal.

7. ¿Qué medicamentos está tomando para la tos?
   No estoy tomando ninguna medicina, pero sí un remedio casero que le tengo mucha fe. Tomo té caliente de limón con miel y también té de orégano. Pero mi hija me dice que necesito tomar medicina.

Recomendaciones

1. Este medicamento puede aliviar los síntomas de la tos que tiene, pero recuerde que no cura la enfermedad. La tos es terca, necesita tiempo para aliviarse completamente. Puede seguir tomando el té de limón con miel si quiere.

2. Esta medicina contiene dos medicamentos. Uno es guaifenesin, un expectorante que le ayuda a hacer la flema más líquida y clara. El otro es dextromethorphan, que le ayuda a controlar la tos.

3. Tome de 1 a 2 cucharaditas de este jarabe cada 4 horas cuando sea necesario para la tos.

Efectos secundarios (molestias)

Le puede causar somnolencia, nerviosismo, irritabilidad o confusión.

Otras recomendaciones

1. No maneje mientras esté tomando esta medicina.
2. Beba mucha agua.

Las preguntas fundamentales[2]

1. ¿Para qué es esta medicina?
   Esta medicina es para calmar la tos.

2. ¿Cómo va a usar esta medicina?
   Voy a tomar de 1 a 2 cucharaditas cada 4 horas cuando sea necesario y debo beber mucha agua.

3. ¿Cuáles son los efectos secundarios?
   Me podría causar somnolencia, nerviosismo, irritabilidad o confusión. Es recomendable no manejar cuando esté tomando este medicamento.

4. Me gustaría ver si le expliqué bien. Por favor, dígame cómo va a usar esta medicina.
   Sí, claro. Por lo general es una medicina muy segura. Es un jarabe para calmar la tos. Voy a tomar de 1 a 2 cucharaditas cada 4 horas cuando sea necesario y puedo seguir tomando el té.

Muy bien, Sra. Huerta. Espero que esta medicina le sirva mucho. Pero si sigue tosiendo, consulte a su doctor.

Ah, muy bien. Gracias por sus recomendaciones, Sra. Chang.

Audio dialogues

PHARMACIST: Good morning. I am Mrs. Chang-Uriarte. I am the pharmacist. Tell me, how can I help you today? How do you feel?

PATIENT: Good morning, Mrs. Chang. My name is Dorotea Huerta. Well, you see, I've had a very stubborn cough. It doesn't go away with anything, not even with oregano or lemon teas. In the evenings, I cough the most; I don't let anyone sleep. What do you recommend that I take?

Questions[1]

1. How long have you had a cough?
   I've had this cough since last weekend.

2. How is the cough? Is it dry or do you have phlegm?
   It's a cough with phlegm.

3. Describe the phlegm.
   Well, it's just phlegm.

   What I mean to say is, what is the consistency? Is it thick or thin? Does it flow easily?
   It's liquid.

   What color is it? Does it have blood? Is it transparent, yellowish, or greenish?
   No, it doesn't have blood. It's clear.

   How much phlegm do you have? Is there a lot or a little?
   I have some phlegm.

4. Does your chest hurt when you cough?
   No, my chest does not hurt, truthfully, but I'm just (already) tired of coughing, because it doesn't let me sleep.

5. Do you smoke?
   No, I do not smoke.

6. Do you have other symptoms?
   No, I don't think so, but I did have a very bad cold a couple weeks ago that I caught from my husband. But I didn't get any bed rest. I kept on working at the store my normal shift.

7. What medications do you take for the cough?
   I am not taking any medicine, but I am taking a home remedy that I have a lot of faith in. I am drinking hot lemon tea with honey and also oregano tea. But my daughter tells me that I need to take medicine.

Recommendations

1. This medication can alleviate the symptoms of your cold, but remember that it will not cure the illness. Coughs may be persis-tent (stubborn). You need time to recuperate completely. You may continue to drink lemon tea with honey if you like.

2. This medicine contains two medications. One is guaifenesin, an expectorant that helps make the phlegm more liquid and clear. The other is dextromethorphan, which helps control (suppress) the cough.

3. Take 1 to 2 teaspoons of this syrup every 4 hours as needed for the cough.

Side effects

It can cause drowsiness, nervousness, irritability, or confusion.

Other recommendations

1. Do not drive while taking this medication.
2. Drink lots of water.

Prime questions[2]

1. What is this medication for?
   This medication is for alleviating the cough.

2. How are you going to use this medication?
   I am going to take 1 to 2 teaspoonfuls every 4 hours as needed, and I should drink a lot of water.

3. What are the side effects?
   It can cause drowsiness, nervousness, irritability, or confusion. It is recommended that I do not drive while I am taking this medicine.

4. I would like to see if I explained it well to you. Please tell me how you are going to use this medicine.
   Yes, of course. For the most part, this medication is safe. This medicine is a syrup to help my cough. I am going to take 1 to 2 teaspoonfuls every 4 hours as needed, and I can continue taking the tea.

Very well, Mrs. Huerta. I hope that this medicine is helpful to you. But if you continue coughing, consult your doctor.

Oh, very well. Thank you for your recommendations, Mrs. Chang.

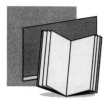

Lección 2   Resfrío
Lesson 2   Cold

Preguntas[1]

1. ¿Qué síntomas tiene?
   – ¿Ha tenido dolor de garganta o tos?
   – ¿Tiene congestión en la nariz o en el pecho? ¿Estornuda frecuentemente?
   – ¿Tiene catarro?
   – ¿Siente escalofríos?
   – ¿Siente malestar general, dolor de cabeza o dolores musculares?
   – ¿Le duelen los pómulos?
2. ¿Desde cuándo tiene estos síntomas?
3. ¿Tiene fiebre?
4. ¿Ha tomado algún medicamento o algún remedio homeopático, naturista o de hierbas?

Recomendaciones

Estos medicamentos no van a curar el resfrío pero pueden aliviar los síntomas.

Para la fiebre: Antipiréticos (aspirina, acetaminofén, ibuprofeno)

Para la tos: Agua, guaifenesín, dextromethorphán

Para el dolor de garganta: Pastillas y trociscos, gárgaras con anestésicos
Gárgaras de phenol al 1.4%
Haga gárgaras con el medicamento durante 15 segundos cada 2 horas.
No las use por más de 2 días.
No se las dé a los niños menores de 12 años sin la recomendación del médico.

Para la congestión: Pseudoephedrine (seudoefedrina) de 30 mg
Tome 1 tableta cada 4 a 6 horas cuando sea necesario (dosis para adultos).
Para comprar este medicamento, necesito ver su identificación. También necesito su firma en esta forma.

Efectos secundarios (molestias)

El medicamento le puede causar las siguientes molestias:
   Corazón: Pulso acelerado, palpitaciones o presión alta.
   También puede sentir insomnio, ansiedad o irritabilidad.

Trociscos de menthol de 5 mg para la tos

Esta medicina le ayuda a calmar el dolor de garganta y la tos.
Chupe 1 trocisco cada 1 o 2 horas, cuando sea necesario.
No los mastique. La medicina se disuelve en la boca.

Otras recomendaciones

1. Lávese frecuentemente las manos.
2. Cúbrase la boca cuando estornude para no contagiar a otras personas.

Las preguntas fundamentales[2]

1. ¿Para qué es esta medicina?
2. ¿Cómo va a usar esta medicina?
3. ¿Cuáles son los efectos secundarios?
4. Me gustaría ver si le expliqué bien. Por favor, dígame cómo va a usar esta medicina.

Questions[1]

1. What are your symptoms?
   - Have you had a sore throat or cough?
   - Do you have congestion in your nose or chest? Do you sneeze frequently?
   - Do you have a runny nose?
   - Do you feel chills?
   - Do you feel general discomfort, headache, or muscle pain?
   - Do your cheekbones (sinuses) hurt?
2. How long have you had these symptoms?
3. Do you have a fever?
4. Have you taken any medication or some homeopathic, natural, or herbal remedy?

Recommendations

These medications are not going to cure the illness, but they can alleviate the symptoms.

For fever: Antipyretics (aspirin, acetaminophen, ibuprofen)

For cough: Water, guaifenesin, dextromethorphan

For sore throat: "Lozenges" and troches, gargles with anesthetic
Phenol gargle (1.4%)
Gargle for 15 seconds every 2 hours.
Don't use it for more than 2 days.
Don't give it to children under 12 years old without the direction of a physician.

For congestion: Pseudoephedrine 30 mg
Take 1 tablet every 4 to 6 hours as needed for congestion (adult dosage).
To buy this medication, I need to see your identification. Also, I need your signature on this form.

Side effects

This medication can cause you the following side effects:
   Heart: Fast pulse, palpitations, or high blood pressure
   You also may experience insomnia, anxiety, or irritability.

Menthol cough drops 5 mg

This medicine helps to relieve sore throat and cough.
Use (Suck on) 1 cough drop every 1 or 2 hours as needed.
Don't chew them. This medicine dissolves in your mouth.

Other recommendations

1. Wash your hands frequently.
2. Cover your mouth when you sneeze so that you don't contaminate other people.

Prime questions[2]

1. What is this medication for?
2. How are you going to use this medication?
3. What are the side effects?
4. I would like to see if I explained it well to you. Please tell me how you are going to use this medicine.

Diálogos para el audio

FARMACÉUTICO: Buenas tardes. Soy el Dr. Samuel Cohen, su farmacéutico. ¿Cómo ha estado?

PACIENTE: *Buenas tardes, doctor. Soy Francisca Aguilar y, pues, ando muy resfriada. Me duele todo el cuerpo. ¿Qué puedo tomar para sentirme mejor? No tengo receta médica. ¿Usted me puede recetar penicilina o algo que me cure rápido?*

FARMACÉUTICO: Lo siento, Sra. Aguilar, pero no la puedo recetar. Solamente los médicos pueden recetar antibióticos. Yo soy farmacéutico. Pero sí puedo recomendarle alguna medicina que no requiera de receta médica y que le va a ayudar a sentirse mejor. Vamos a ver. Necesito hacerle algunas preguntas.

Preguntas[1]

1. ¿Qué síntomas tiene? ¿Ha tenido dolor de garganta o tos?
   Sí, he tenido dolor de garganta, pero no muy fuerte, desde anteayer.

   ¿Tiene congestión en la nariz o en el pecho? ¿Estornuda frecuentemente? ¿Tiene catarro?
   Tengo congestión en la nariz y estornudo con frecuencia. Traigo mucho catarro.

   ¿Siente escalofríos?
   A veces siento escalofríos.

   ¿Siente malestar general, dolor de cabeza o dolores musculares?
   Como le dije, me duele todo el cuerpo y también me duele la cabeza.

   ¿Le duelen los pómulos?
   Un poco, pero no tanto.

2. ¿Desde cuándo tiene estos síntomas?
   Desde hace 2 días.

3. ¿Tiene fiebre?
   Bueno no sé, me siento algo caliente, pero no me he tomado la temperatura.

4. ¿Ha tomado algún medicamento o algún remedio homeopático, naturista o de hierbas?
   Ahora mismo, no.

Recomendaciones

1. Estos medicamentos no van a curarle el resfrío, pero pueden aliviar los síntomas. También, lávese seguido las manos. Cúbrase la boca cuando estornude para no contagiar a otras personas.
2. Para la fiebre o los dolores musculares puede tomar cualquier antipirético: aspirina, ibuprofeno o acetaminofén.

¿Tiene presión alta?
No, no tengo alta presión.

Entonces, para la congestión le voy a recomendar seudoefedrina de 30 mg. Tome 1 tableta cada 4 a 6 horas cuando sea necesario. Para comprar este medicamento, necesito ver su identificación. También necesito su firma en esta forma, por favor.

Efectos secundarios (molestias)

1. Esta medicine le puede causar las siguientes molestias. Podría tener pulso acelerado o una subida en su presión. También puede sentir insomnio, ansiedad o irritabilidad.
2. Para el dolor de garganta le voy a recomendar estos trociscos. Le van a ayudar a calmar la irritación en la garganta. Chupe un trocisco cada 1 a 2 horas. No lo mastique. La medicina va a disolverse en la boca.
3. Si no quiere el trocisco, haga gárgaras de agua con sal si gusta para calmar el dolor de garganta.

Las preguntas fundamentales[2]

1. ¿Para qué es esta medicina?
   Una de las recomendaciones es seudoefedrina para la congestión. Y para la irritación en la garganta voy a hacer gárgaras de agua con sal cuando quiera o voy a chupar uno de estos trociscos cada 1 a 2 horas. Para el malestar general o la febrícula, puedo tomar acetaminofén.

   Sí, muy bien.

2. Ahora, ¿Cómo va a usar la seudoefedrina?
   Voy a tomar 1 tableta cada 4 a 6 horas sólo cuando sea necesario.

3. ¿Cuáles son los efectos secundarios de la seudoefedrina?
   Puede afectar lu presión o también provocar pulso acelerado. Puedo sentir irritabilidad, ansiedad o insomnio.

4. Me gustaría ver si le expliqué bien. Por favor, dígame cómo va a usar esta medicina.
   Sí, claro. Para la congestión voy a tomar 1 tableta de seudoefedrina cada 4 a 6 horas sólo cuando sea necesario. Y para el dolor de garganta voy a hacer gárgaras de agua con sal cuando quiera o voy a chupar 1 trocisco cada 1 a 2 horas. Para el malestar general o la febrícula, puedo tomar acetaminofén.

Muy bien, Sra. Aguilar, creo que entendió bien las instrucciones. Si no se siente mejor en unos días o los síntomas empeoran, es recomendable que consulte a su médico. Esperamos que se sienta mejor.

Muchas gracias, doctor. Hasta luego.

■ *Audio dialogues*

PHARMACIST: Good afternoon. My name is Dr. Samuel Cohen, your pharmacist. How have you been?

PATIENT: *Good afternoon, Doctor. I am Francisca Aguilar and, well, I have had a bad cold. My whole body aches. What can I take to feel better? I don't have a prescription. Can you prescribe penicillin or something that can cure me fast?*

PHARMACIST: I'm sorry, Mrs. Aguilar, but I cannot prescribe it. Only a medical doctor can prescribe antibiotics. I am a pharmacist. Nevertheless, I can recommend a medicine that doesn't require a prescription and that may help you feel better. Let's see. I need to ask you a few questions.

Questions[1]

1. What are your symptoms? Have you had a sore throat or cough?
   Yes, I've had a sore throat, but not too bad, since the day before yesterday.

   Do you have congestion in your nose or chest? Do you sneeze very often? Do you have a runny nose?
   I have nasal congestion, and I sneeze often. I have a very runny nose.

   Do you feel chills?
   Sometimes I have chills.

   Do you feel general discomfort, headache, or muscle pain?
   As I explained to you, I have body aches, and also my head hurts

   Do your cheekbones (sinuses) hurt?
   A little, but not much.

2. How long have you had these symptoms?
   Since 2 days ago.

3. Do you have a fever?
   I don't really know. I feel slightly warm, but I have not taken my temperature.

4. Have you taken any medication or some homeopathic, natural, or herbal remedy?
   No, not right now.

Recommendations

1. These medications are not going to cure the cold, but they can alleviate the symptoms. Also, wash your hands continuously. Cover your mouth when you sneeze so that you don't contaminate other people.
2. For the fever or muscle pain, you can take any antipyretic: aspirin, ibuprofen, or acetaminophen.

Do you have high blood pressure?
No, I don't have high blood pressure.

Then, for the congestion, I am going to recommend pseudoephedrine 30 mg. Take 1 tablet every 4 to 6 hours as needed. To buy this medicine, I need to see your identification. Also, I need your signature on this form, please.

Side effects

1. This medicine can cause you the following effects. You could have a fast pulse or a rise in your blood pressure. You also may experience insomnia, anxiety, or irritability.
2. For the sore throat, I am going to recommend these troches (cough drops). They are going to help relieve the irritation in your throat. Suck on a drop every 1 to 2 hours. Don't chew it. The medicine will dissolve in your mouth.
3. If you don't want the cough drop, gargle with water and salt, if you like, to relieve the sore throat.

Prime questions[2]

1. What is this medication for?
   One of the recommendations is pseudoephedrine for congestion. And for the throat irritation, I am going to gargle with water and salt when I like, or I am going to suck on one of these drops every 1 to 2 hours. For the general malaise (body aches) or slight fever, I can take acetaminophen.

   Yes, very good.

2. Now, how are you going to use the pseudoephedrine?
   I am going to take 1 tablet every 4 to 6 hours only when it's necessary.

3. What are the side effects of pseudoephedrine?
   It can affect the blood pressure or also provoke a fast pulse. I can feel irritability, anxiety, or insomnia.

4. I would like to see if I explained it well to you. Please tell me how you are going to use this medicine.
   Yes, of course. For the congestion, I am going to take 1 tablet of pseudoephedrine every 4 to 6 hours only when it is necessary. And for the sore throat, I am going to gargle with water and salt when I like, or I am going to suck on 1 of these drops every 1 to 2 hours. For the general bad feeling or slight fever, I can take acetaminophen.

Very well, Mrs. Aguilar, I think that you understand the instructions well. If you don't feel better in a few days, or if the symptoms worsen, it's recommended that you consult your doctor. We hope you feel better.

Thank you very much, Doctor. Until later.

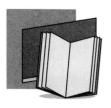

Lección 3   Alergias al medio ambiente
Lesson 3   Seasonal allergies

Preguntas[1]

1. ¿Qué síntomas tiene?
   - ¿Tiene los ojos llorosos o enrojecidos?
   - ¿Tiene irritación en la nariz o los ojos?
   - ¿Ha tenido catarro? ¿Estornuda mucho?
   - ¿Tiene congestión nasal o la nariz tapada?
2. ¿Desde cuándo tiene estos síntomas?
3. ¿Está tomando otros medicamentos?

Recomendaciones
Loratadine de 10 mg (antihistamínico)
Tome 1 pastilla a diario con el estómago vacío cuando sea necesario para las alergias.

Efectos secundarios (molestias)
El medicamento le puede provocar somnolencia, dolor de cabeza o boca seca.

Las preguntas fundamentales[2]

1. ¿Para qué es esta medicina?
2. ¿Cómo va a tomar esta medicina?
3. ¿Cuales son los efectos secundarios?
4. Me gustaría ver si le expliqué bien. Por favor, dígame cómo va a usar esta medicina.

Questions[1]

1. What are your symptoms?
   – Do you have teary or reddened eyes?
   – Are your nose or eyes irritated?
   – Have you had a runny nose? Do you sneeze a lot?
   – Do you have nasal congestion or a "stopped up" nose?
2. How long have you had these symptoms?
3. Are you taking any other medicines?

Recommendations:

Loratadine 10 mg (antihistamine)
Take 1 tablet daily on an empty stomach as needed for allergies.

Side effects

This medication can cause drowsiness, headaches, or dry mouth.

Prime questions[2]

1. What is this medication for?
2. How are you going to take this medication?
3. What are the side effects?
4. I would like to see if I explained it well to you. Please tell me how you are going to use this medicine.

Diálogos para el audio

FARMACÉUTICA: Buenas tardes. Soy la Dra. Sánchez. Dígame, ¿en qué le puedo ayudar?

PACIENTE: *Doctora, buenas tardes. Mi nombre es Diana Pérez. Ay, pues, fíjese que tengo muchas molestias. No sé si es gripe, resfrío, o si son alergias. ¡Estornudo mucho! (¡Ahhhh-chooo!) Discúlpeme pero estornudo siempre con mucha fuerza. ¿Qué puedo tomar para que se me quite tanta molestia?*

FARMACÉUTICA: Pues, vamos a ver, Sra. Pérez. Antes de recomendarle algún producto necesito hacerle algunas preguntas.

PACIENTE: *Sí, claro, entiendo.*

Preguntas[1]

1. ¿Qué síntomas tiene? ¿Cómo se siente?
   Pues, últimamente, no muy bien con tantos malestares.

2. Lo siento. ¿Tiene los ojos llorosos o enrojecidos?
   Sí, he tenido los ojos muy llorosos y enrojecidos desde ayer así como me los ve ahorita. Traigo hasta la vista borrosa.

3. ¿Tiene irritación en la nariz o en los ojos? ¿Tiene comezón o picazón en los ojos?
   Sí, tengo mucha irritación en la nariz, algo de carraspera, y tengo comezón en los ojos.

4. ¿Ha tenido catarro? ¿Ha estado estornudando muy frecuentemente?
   No, no he tenido mucho catarro, pero estoy estornudando mucho, especialmente cuando estoy fuera de mi casa.

5. ¿Tiene congestión nasal o nariz tapada?
   Ahora no.

6. ¿Desde cuándo tiene estos síntomas?
   Desde hace una semana me siento mal. Es primavera y batallo con el polen. Me molesta mucho.

Pues, parece que tiene algunos de los síntomas clásicos de las alergias. Por ahora, voy a recomendarle esta medicina para aliviar esos síntomas. Pero si sigue con molestias, es mejor que consulte a su médico.

Recomendaciones

Esta medicina se llama loratadina y es un antihistamínico. Tome una pastilla de 10 mg a diario con el estómago vacío cuando sea necesario para las alergias.

Efectos secundarios (molestias)

El medicamento le puede provocar somnolencia, dolor de cabeza o boca seca.

Las preguntas fundamentales[2]

1. ¿Para qué es esta medicina?
   Esta medicina es para aliviar los síntomas de las alergias. Es un antihistamínico.

2. ¿Cómo va a tomar esta medicina?
   Puedo tomar 1 pastilla diariamente con el estómago vacío cuando sea necesario.

3. ¿Cuales son los efectos secundarios?
   El medicamento me puede provocar somnolencia, dolor de cabeza o boca seca.

4. Me gustaría ver si le expliqué bien. Por favor, dígame cómo va a usar esta medicina.
   Sí, claro. La medicina se llama loratadina. Puedo tomar 1 pastilla cada día para los síntomas de alergias.

Muy bien. Espero que se sienta mejor, Sra. Perez. Adiós.

Audio dialogues

PHARMACIST: Good afternoon. I am Dr. Sánchez. Tell me, how can I help you?

PATIENT: *Doctor, good afternoon. My name is Diana Pérez. Oh, you see, I feel lousy. I do not know if I have the flu, a cold, or allergies. I've been sneezing a lot! (Ahhhh-chooo!) I apologize, but I sneeze rather loudly. What can I take to get rid of these bothersome (symptoms)?*

PHARMACIST: Well, let's see, Mrs. Pérez. Before recommending a product, I need to ask you a few questions.

PATIENT: *Yes, of course, I understand.*

Questions[1]

1. What are your symptoms? How do you feel?
   Well, lately not very well with all of these discomforts (symptoms).

2. I'm sorry to hear that. Do you have teary or red eyes?
   Yes, I have had very teary and reddened eyes since yesterday, just like you see them now. I even carry (have) blurry vision.

3. Is your nose or eyes irritated? Do your eyes itch?
   Yes, my nose is very irritated, I am somewhat hoarse, and my eyes are itchy.

4. Have you had a runny nose? Have you been sneezing a lot?
   No, I have not had much of a runny nose, but I am sneezing a lot, especially when I go outside my house.

5. Do you have nasal congestion or a "stopped up" nose?
   Right now, no.

6. How long have you had these symptoms?
   For about a week, I have felt bad. It is springtime, and I have a hard time (battle) with the pollen. It bothers me a lot.

Well, it looks like you have some of the classic symptoms of allergies. For now, I am going to recommend this medication to alleviate those symptoms. But if you continue with these symptoms, it is better that you consult your doctor.

Recommendations

This medicine, which is called loratadine, is an antihistamine. Take one 10 mg tablet daily on an empty stomach when it's necessary for your allergies.

Side effects

This medication can cause drowsiness, headaches, or dry mouth.

Prime questions[2]

1. What is this medication for?
   This medicine is to treat allergy symptoms. It is an antihistamine.

2. How are you going to use this medication?
   I can take 1 tablet daily on an empty stomach as needed.

3. What are the side effects?
   The medication can cause drowsiness, headaches, or dry mouth.

4. I would like to see if I explained it well to you. Please tell me how you are going to use this medicine.
   Yes, of course. The medicine is called loratadine. I can take 1 tablet every day for allergy symptoms.

Very good. I hope that you feel better, Mrs. Pérez. Goodbye.

De la cultura / About the culture

1. Common treatments for cough in the Hispanic culture include drinking hot tea with lemon, taking honey with lemon, and putting hot compresses over the patient's chest and back.

2. Common treatments for cold in the Hispanic culture include the following:
   a. Apply ointments containing menthol, eucalyptus, or both to the patient's chest and back.
   b. Immerse the patient's feet in hot water for a few minutes, and have the patient lie in bed with many blankets to make him or her sweat profusely.
   c. Have the patient drink lots of hot beverages (mainly herbal teas with lime and honey).

3. Beliefs in some Hispanic cultures suggest that colds may be caused by walking barefoot on a cold floor. This explanation is similar to the saying in the United States, "Don't go outside with your hair wet or you'll catch a cold."

4. The following are some expressions not in the vocabulary but used commonly in certain Latin American countries:
   a. "**guardar cama**"—meaning "to stay in bed all day due to illness"
   b. "**remedios caseros**"—meaning "home remedies"
   c. "**carraspera**"—meaning "hoarseness"

5. The idiomatic expression "**batallar con**" is used to say "to battle or fight with" a symptom, infection, disease, or medication. It describes a situation in which you are "fighting with" something that is bothersome. For example, "**Batallo con esta medicina—es muy amarga**" means "I am fighting to take this medicine—it is very bitter."

6. Patients often use the conjugated verb "**traer**" to describe that they are "carrying" a problem, illness, or feeling. For example, "**Traigo mucha tos**," "**Traigo mucha hambre**," and "**Traemos muchos problemas**" mean, respectively, "I have (am carrying) a lot of coughing," "I am (carrying) very hungry," and "We have (are carrying) a lot of problems."

7. The term "**trocisco**" in Spanish is a more technical term for "cough drops." Regional variations for "cough drops" will exist. One example used on the U.S.–Mexico border is "**dulce**."

Apuntes de gramática / Grammar notes

Present perfect

Example:	(haber + past participle)	<u>He tenido</u> fiebre desde ayer.
	(have + past participle)	I <u>have had</u> a fever since yesterday.

Some irregular verbs in past participle

Example: (infinitive—past participle)

abrir—abierto
cubrir—cubierto
decir—dicho
escribir—escrito
hacer—hecho
poner—puesto
ver—visto
volver—vuelto

Present progressive

Example:	(estar + "gerundio")	Mi hijo <u>está llorando</u>.
	(is + present participle)	My son <u>is crying</u>.

Ejercicios / Exercises

I. Haga una pregunta para cada respuesta. (Write a question for each answer.)

1. ¿_____?
   Es seca.

2. ¿_____?
   He tosido más durante la noche.

3. ¿_____?
   Desde hace dos días.

4. ¿_____?
   No, no he tomado nada, sólo he estado bebiendo muchos tés.

II. Llene los espacios en blanco con los verbos conjugados o las palabras correctas. (Fill in the blanks with the conjugated verbs or correct words.)

1. *Paciente:* Siento un malestar general. Desde ayer (haber, estar) ____ _____ resfriado. Tengo
   _____, _____ y _____.

2. **Farmacéutica:** (Describir) _____ cómo se siente cuando (toser)_____.

3. *Paciente:* Cuando (toser) _____, siento dolor en el pecho y (tener) _____ flema. La flema (ser)
   _____ y (contener) _____ sangre.

4. **Farmacéutica:** (Tener que, consultar) _____ _____ _____ a su doctor.

III. Escoja las palabras que correspondan al inglés. (Select the word that corresponds to the English translation.)

____ 1. los escalofríos   a. dry

____ 2. el estornudo   b. reddened

____ 3. el catarro   c. thick

____ 4. lloroso(a)   d. chills

____ 5. enrojecido(a)   e. tearful

____ 6. la nariz tapada   f. runny nose

____ 7. espeso(a)   g. loose

____ 8. flojo(a)   h. itchiness

____ 9. la picazón   i. "stopped up" nose

____10. seco(a)   j. sneeze

IV. Verbos. Escriba oraciones usando el participio pasado (presente perfecto) o el gerundio (presente progresivo).
(Write sentences using the past participle [present perfect] or gerund [present progressive].)

1. Haber + escribir / Estar + escribir

2. Haber + toser / Estar + toser

3. Haber + ver / Estar + ver

4. Haber + hacer / Estar + hacer

5. Haber + poner / Estar + poner

6. Haber + volver / Estar + volver

7. Haber + ir / Estar + ir

8. Haber + abrir / Estar + abrir

9. Haber + cubrir / Estar + cubrir

10. Haber + decir / Estar + decir

11. Haber + quitar / Estar + quitar

V. Busque en el Internet un sitio en español y escriba un párrafo sobre uno de los siguientes temas.
(Look up an Internet site in Spanish and write a paragraph about one of the following topics.)

1. las enfermedades con mucha tos (e.g., tuberculosis, tosferina)

2. la diferencia entre resfrío y gripe

3. las causas de las alergias

4. la sinusitis

REFERENCES

1. Tietze KJ. Cough. In: Berardi RR, Kroon LA, McDermott JH, et al., eds. *Handbook of Nonprescription Drugs.* 15th ed. Washington, DC: American Pharmacists Association; 2006:229–42.
2. Gardner M, Boyce RW, Herrier RN. *Pharmacist–Patient Consultation Program PPCP-Unit I: An Interactive Approach to Verifying Patient Understanding.* New York: Pfizer Educational Services; 1991.

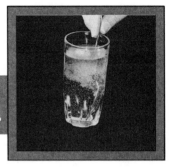

Capítulo
Chapter 4

Estreñimiento y diarrea
Constipation and diarrhea

Verbos / Verbs		Presente / Present tense			
		Yo	Él, ella, usted	Mandato	Ejemplos
bajar	to go down, to lower, to lose (weight)	bajo	baja	Baje	*Baje de peso.*
comenzar	to begin, to start	comienzo	comienza	Comience	*Comience hoy el tratamiento.*
comer	to eat	como	come	Coma	*Coma porciones más pequeñas.*
dar	to give	doy	da	Dé(le)	*Déle suero oral a su niño.*
esperar	to wait	espero	espera	Espere	*Espere 5 minutos antes de tomar otra medicina.*
estimular	to stimulate	estimulo	estimula	Estimule	*Estimule su intestino comiendo fibra.*
explicar	to explain	explico	explica	Explique(me)	*Explíqueme su problema.*
facilitar	to facilitate	facilito	facilita	Facilite	*La medicina facilita la evacuación.*
funcionar	to function	funciono	funciona	Funcione	*La medicina no me funciona para la diarrea.*
mezclar	to mix	mezclo	mezcla	Mezcle	*Mezcle esta medicina con agua.*
notar	to notice	noto	nota	Note	*¿Nota algún cambio en su salud?*
pensar	to think	pienso	piensa	Piense	*Piense en hacer un cambio de hábitos.*
perder	to lose	pierdo	pierde	Pierda	*No pierda la receta.*
quejar(se)	to complain	me quejo	se queja	Quéjese	*El niño se queja de dolor.*
regir	to move the bowels	rijo	rige	Rija	*Rija siempre a la misma hora.*
salir	to go out, to leave	salgo	sale	Salga	*Salga por la puerta de enfrente.*
suavizar	to soften	suavizo	suaviza	Suavice	*La medicina suaviza los excrementos.*
tratar	to try, to treat (illness)	trato	trata	Trate	*La doctora trata el estreñimiento con este laxante.*
viajar	to travel	viajo	viaja	Viaje	*¿Qué tan seguido viaja?*

El sistema digestivo (parte baja) / Digestive system (lower portion)

el ano	anus
el colon	colon
el intestino delgado	small intestine
el intestino grueso	large intestine
el recto	rectum

Sustantivos / Nouns

la alimentación	usual diet
el apetito	appetite
el baño	bathroom, bath
la bolsa	bag
el caldo	clear broth
el cambio	change
la cápsula	capsule
la causa	cause
el cólico	abdominal cramp
el color	color
la comida	meal
la confusión	confusion
la debilidad	weakness
la dificultad	difficulty
el dolor abdominal	abdominal pain
el ejercicio	exercise
el estreñimiento	constipation
la evacuación	bowel movement
el excremento	excrement, stools
la fibra	fiber
la forma	form
la frecuencia	frequency
la fruta	fruit
las heces fecales	stools
la hierba	herb
la incomodidad	discomfort
la infusión	infusion
el jugo	juice
el laxante	laxative
las legumbres	legumes
el líquido	liquid
el moco	mucus
el momento	moment
el país	country
la palabra	word
el pan integral	whole-grain bread
la pérdida	loss
la pipí (euphemism)	urine
el polvo	powder, dust
la popó (euphemism)	feces, stools
el problema	problem
el remedio	remedy
la sed	thirst
la soltura (euphemism)	diarrhea
el suero oral	oral rehydration
el tiempo	time
el tratamiento	treatment
las verduras, los vegetales	vegetables

Adjetivos / Adjectives

aguado(a)	watery
débil	weak
desgrasado(a)	without fat
diferente	different
duro(a)	hard
menor	minor
normal	normal
persistente	persistent
propio(a)	own
reseco(a)	dry
turístico(a)	tourist-like

Otras expresiones / Other expressions

a veces	sometimes
actualmente	currently
adentro	inside of
antes	before
¿Desde cuándo?	Since when?
durante	during
hacer del cuerpo (euphemism)	to go to the bathroom (stool)
hacer del dos (euphemism)	to move the bowels
hacer ejercicio	to exercise
ir al baño	to go to the bathroom
obstrucción intestinal	intestinal obstruction
perder el apetito	to lose appetite
¿Qué tan seguido?	How often?
tener dificultad para	to have a hard time
tener edad ___	to be ___ years old
tener sed	to be thirsty (to have thirst)
últimamente	lately
usualmente	usually

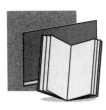

Lección 1 Estreñimiento
Lesson 1 Constipation

Preguntas[1]

1. ¿Por cuánto tiempo ha estado estreñido?
2. ¿Qué tan seguido va al baño (hace del cuerpo)? ¿Va al baño menos o más de lo normal?
3. ¿Está rigiendo diferente de lo usual? ¿Ha tenido cambios en los excrementos? ¿Por ejemplo, son duros o suaves?
4. ¿Las heces han cambiado de color o de forma? ¿Hay sangre? Explíqueme los cambios.
5. ¿Tiene dolor o molestias cuando va al baño?
6. ¿Qué otros problemas ha tenido? Por ejemplo: ¿Tiene dolor de estómago? ¿Náusea o vómito? ¿Incomodidad? ¿Pérdida de peso? ¿Inflamación abdominal?
7. ¿Ha tenido cambios en su alimentación? ¿Por ejemplo, come más cereales, más pan integral o más frutas y verduras?
8. ¿Hace ejercicio? ¿Cuánto? ¿Con qué frecuencia?
9. ¿Durante el día, cuántos vasos de agua o de otros líquidos toma?
10. ¿Ha usado laxantes, té o remedios de hierbas para este problema? ¿Qué tan seguido usa laxantes? ¿Desde cuándo los usa?
11. ¿Tiene alguna molestia cuando usa los laxantes? ¿Por ejemplo, tiene diarrea o dolor de estómago?

Recomendaciones

1. Docusate 50 mg

Tome 1 cápsula cada 6 horas cuando sea necesario. Esta medicina suaviza los excrementos y facilita la evacuación.

Efectos secundarios (molestias)

Puede causar cólicos y diarrea.

2. Psyllium (3.4 g / 1 cucharada)

Mezcle una cucharada de este polvo en un vaso de agua.
Puede tomar la medicina de una a tres veces al día cuando sea necesario.
A veces va a necesitar de 2 a 3 días para que la medicina funcione.
Esta medicina es como fibra y funciona en sus intestinos.
Espere de 2 a 3 horas antes de tomar otras medicinas.

Efectos secundarios (molestias)

Puede causar cólicos, diarrea u obstrucción intestinal.

3. Té o infusión de hojas de sen (20 mg / 1 bolsa de té)

Esta hierba ayuda a estimular el movimiento de los intestinos.
Ponga una bolsa de té en agua caliente. Tome una taza antes de acostarse. No contiene cafeína.
No lo use en niños menores de 6 años.

Las preguntas fundamentales[2]

1. ¿Para qué es esta medicina?
2. ¿Cómo va a usar esta medicina?
3. ¿Cuáles son los efectos secundarios?
4. Me gustaría ver si le expliqué bien. Por favor, dígame cómo va a usar esta medicina.

Questions[1]

1. How long have you been constipated?
2. How often do you have a bowel movement? Do you go to the bathroom less or more often than usual?
3. Are you having different bowel movements than usual? Have you had changes in your stools? For example, are they hard or soft?
4. Have the stools changed in color or shape? Is there blood? Explain to me the changes.
5. Do you have pain or trouble (bothersome effects) when you go to the bathroom?
6. What other problems have you had? For example: Do you have stomach pain? Nausea or vomiting? Discomfort? Weight loss? Bloating?
7. Has there been a change in your diet? For example: Do you eat more cereal, more whole-grain bread, or more fruit and vegetables?
8. Do you exercise? How much? How often?
9. During the day, how many glasses of water or other liquids do you drink?
10. Have you used laxatives, teas, or herbal remedies for this problem? How often do you use laxatives? Since when have you used laxatives?
11. Do you have other effects when you use laxatives? For example, do you have diarrhea or stomachache?

Recommendations

1. Docusate 50 mg

Take 1 capsule every 6 hours as needed. This medication makes the stool softer and helps to facilitate a bowel movement (evacuation).

Side effects

It may cause abdominal cramping and diarrhea.

2. Psyllium (3.4 g / 1 tablespoonful)

Mix a tablespoonful of the powder with a glass of water.
You can take the medicine one to three times a day as needed.
Sometimes you will need 2 to 3 days for the medication to work.
This medication is like fiber and works in the intestines.
Wait 2 to 3 hours before taking other medication.

Side effects

It may cause abdominal cramping, diarrhea, or intestinal obstruction.

3. Senna leaf tea (20 mg / 1 teabag)

This herb helps to stimulate the movement of the intestines.
Put a teabag in hot water. Drink the cup of tea before going to bed. It does not contain caffeine.
Do not use in children under 6 years of age.

Prime questions[2]

1. What is this medication for?
2. How are you going to use this medication?
3. What are the side effects?
4. I would like to see if I explained it well to you. Please tell me how you are going to use this medicine.

Diálogos para el audio

FARMACÉUTICA: Buenas tardes. Soy la Dra. White. ¿En qué le puedo servir?

PACIENTE: *Buenas tardes, doctora. Soy Ernesto Martínez. Sabe que estoy muy estreñido y me siento muy mal. Quisiera que me recomendara alguna medicina para este problema.*

FARMACÉUTICA: Sí, como no. Pero primero quiero hacerle unas preguntas.

PACIENTE: *Por supuesto, doctora.*

Preguntas[1]

1. ¿Por cuánto tiempo ha estado estreñido?
   No he podido ir al baño desde hace 3 días.

2. ¿Qué tan seguido va al baño? ¿Va al baño menos o más de lo normal?
   Siempre tengo algo de problema para ir al baño, pero generalmente voy una vez al día, por las mañanas. Pero estos días no he podido regir.

3. ¿Está rigiendo diferente de lo usual? ¿Ha tenido cambios en los excrementos? ¿Por ejemplo, son duros o suaves?
   Ahora son muy duros.

4. ¿Las heces han cambiado de color o de forma? ¿Hay sangre? Explíqueme los cambios.
   Pues, son muy gruesos y muy duros. Además, sólo puedo regir muy poco. Pero no he notado sangre en los excrementos.

5. ¿Tiene dolor o molestias cuando va al baño?
   Sí, me duele mucho el recto cuando hago el esfuerzo de regir.

6. ¿Qué otros problemas ha tenido? Por ejemplo: ¿Tiene dolor de estómago? ¿Náusea o vómito? ¿Incomodidad? ¿Pérdida de peso? ¿Inflamación abdominal?
   No tengo dolor de estómago, pero siento un poco de náusea. También estoy muy incómodo y todo el tiempo me siento muy inflamado del estómago. Pero creo que no he bajado de peso.

7. ¿Ha tenido cambios en su alimentación? ¿Por ejemplo, come más cereales, más pan integral o más frutas y verduras?
   No, generalmente no como frutas ni verduras y nada más como cereales de caja.

8. ¿Hace ejercicio? ¿Cuánto? ¿Con qué frecuencia?
   Nunca hago ejercicio. De vez en cuando camino cuando voy al centro comercial.

9. ¿Durante el día, cuántos vasos de agua o de otros líquidos toma?
   Nunca tomo agua porque no me gusta. Pero me tomo como dos o tres refrescos al día.

10. ¿Ha usado laxantes, té o remedios de hierbas para este problema? ¿Qué tan seguido usa laxantes? ¿Desde cuándo los usa?
    Tomo el té de hojas de sen para este problema, pero ya no me hace efecto.

11. ¿Tiene alguna molestia cuando usa los laxantes? ¿Por ejemplo, tiene diarrea o dolor de estómago?
    No, siempre me ayudaba el té para el estreñimiento, pero últimamente no me ha funcionado.

Recomendaciones

1. Bueno, le voy a recomendar una medicina muy efectiva para este problema. Se llama psyllium y es un polvo. Úselo de la siguiente manera: Mezcle 1 cucharada de este polvo en un vaso de agua.

2. Puede tomarlo de una a tres veces al día cuando sea necesario.

3. A veces va a necesitar de 2 a 3 días para que la medicina funcione.

4. Esta medicina es como fibra y funciona en sus intestinos.

5. Espere de 2 a 3 horas antes de tomar otras medicinas.

Efectos secundarios (molestias)

Esta medicina puede causarle cólicos, diarrea u obstrucción intestinal.

Las preguntas fundamentales[2]

Repítame las instrucciones, por favor.

1. ¿Para qué es esta medicina?
   Para el estreñimiento.

2. ¿Cómo va a usar esta medicina?
   Voy a mezclar 1 cucharada de este polvo en un vaso de agua. Pero no me acuerdo cuantas veces al día.

   Va a tomarla de una a tres veces al día, si es necesario.
   Ah, sí.

3. ¿Cuáles son los efectos secundarios?
   Puedo tener cólicos o diarrea.

4. Me gustaría ver si le expliqué bien. Por favor, dígame cómo va a usar esta medicina.
   Voy a disolver 1 cucharada de este polvo en un vaso con agua y voy a tomarlo de una a tres veces al día, si es necesario.

Muy bien. Espero que se le quite el estreñimiento. Pero si no se le quita, consulte a su doctor.

Muchas gracias, doctora. Que Dios la bendiga.

Gracias, igualmente.

■ *Audio dialogues*

PHARMACIST: Good afternoon. I am Dr. White. How can I help you?

PATIENT: *Good afternoon, Doctor. I am Ernesto Martínez. You know, I am very constipated and I feel bad. I would like for you to recommend to me some medicine for this problem.*

PHARMACIST: Yes, of course. But first I want to ask you a few questions.

PATIENT: *Of course, Doctor.*

Questions[1]

1. How long have you been constipated?
    I haven't been able to go to the bathroom for 3 days.

2. How often do you go to the bathroom? Do you go to the bathroom less or more often than usual?
    I always have problems going to the bathroom, but generally I go once a day, in the mornings. These days I haven't been able to move my bowels (to go).

3. Are you having different bowel movements than usual? Have you had changes in your stools? For example, are they hard or soft?
    Right now, they are very hard.

4. Have the stools changed in color or shape? Is there blood? Explain to me the changes.
    Well, they are very thick and hard. Besides, I only go very little. But I haven't noticed blood in the stools.

5. Do you have pain or trouble (bothersome effects) when you go to the bathroom?
    Yes, the rectum hurts me a lot when I make the effort to go to the bathroom (have a bowel movement).

6. What other problems have you had? For example: Do you have stomach pain? Nausea or vomiting? Discomfort? Weight loss? Abdominal bloating?
    I don't have stomach pain, but I have a little nausea. Also, I am very uncomfortable, and I am bloated all of the time. However, I think that I have not lost weight.

7. Has there been a change in your diet? For example, do you eat more cereal, more whole-grain bread, or more fruit and vegetables?
    No, I generally don't eat fruits or vegetables, and I only eat cold (boxed) cereals.

8. Do you exercise? How much? How often?
    No, I never exercise. I walk once in a while when I go to the mall.

9. During the day, how many glasses of water or other liquids do you drink?
    I never drink water because I don't like it. But I drink two or three sodas a day.

10. Have you used laxatives, teas, or herbal remedies for this problem? How often do you use laxatives? Since when have you used laxatives?

I drink a tea from senna leaf for this problem, but it doesn't work for me any more (it no longer makes any effect on me).

11. Do you have other problems when you use laxatives? For example, do you have diarrhea or stomachache?
    No, the tea always helped me for this problem, but lately it doesn't work (function) for me.

Recommendations

1. Well, I am going to recommend a medicine for you that is very effective for this problem. It is called psyllium, and it is a powder. Use it in the following way: Mix 1 tablespoonful of the powder in a glass of water.
2. You can take it one to three times a day when it is needed.
3. Sometimes you will need 2 to 3 days for the medication will work.
4. This medication is like fiber and works in the intestines.
5. Wait 2 to 3 hours before taking other medication.

Side effects

This medicine may cause abdominal cramping, diarrhea, or intestinal obstruction.

Prime questions[2]

Repeat the directions for me, please.

1. What is this medication for?
    For constipation.

2. How are you going to use this medication?
    I am going to mix 1 tablespoonful of the powder in a glass of water. But I don't remember how many times a day.

    You are going to take it one to three times a day, if it is necessary.
    Oh, yes.

3. What are the side effects?
    I can have abdominal cramping or diarrhea.

4. I would like to see if I explained it well to you. Please tell me how you are going to use this medicine.
    I am going to mix 1 tablespoonful of the powder in a glass of water, and I am going to take it one to three times a day if needed.

Very good. I hope that you get rid of your constipation. But if you don't get rid of it, consult your doctor.

Thank you, Doctor. God bless you.

Thank you. Likewise.

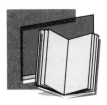

Lección 2   Diarrea
Lesson 2   Diarrhea

Preguntas[3]
Para el adulto

1. ¿Desde cuándo ha tenido diarrea?
2. ¿Cuántas veces al día va al baño?

3. Por favor, describa los excrementos: ¿Son aguados o líquidos? ¿Hay sangre o moco?

4. ¿Tuvo cambios en la comida?
5. ¿Ha viajado en los últimos días? ¿Salió fuera del país?
6. ¿Qué medicamentos o remedios de hierbas toma? ¿Está tomando algún antibiótico?
7. ¿Ha tenido otras molestias?

8. ¿Tiene fiebre?
9. ¿Tiene sed o siente la boca reseca?
10. ¿Tiene dolor de estómago, cólicos, vómito o pérdida del apetito?
11. ¿Ha tenido mareos, confusión, irritabilidad o debilidad?

Para el niño
¿Cuántos años tiene su hijo(a)?
1. ¿Desde cuándo tiene diarrea su niño(a)?
2. ¿Cuántas evacuaciones tuvo? ¿Cuántas veces fue al baño?
3. Por favor dígame cómo son los excrementos del niño (de la niña): ¿Son aguados o líquidos? ¿Tienen sangre o moco?
4. ¿Comió algo diferente?
5. ¿Ha ido a otra casa? ¿Lo ha llevado de viaje?
6. ¿Le está dando alguna medicina o algún remedio de hierbas? ¿Le está dando algún antibiótico?
7. ¿Le ha notado otros síntomas aparte de la soltura (diarrea)?
8. ¿Tiene fiebre?
9. ¿Tiene sed o le nota la boca muy reseca?
10. ¿Se ha quejado de dolor de estómago, cólicos, o ha perdido el apetito?
11. ¿Ha notado que esté mareado, irritable o muy débil? ¿Ha tenido síntomas de confusión?

Recomendaciones
Loperamide 2 mg (para adulto)
1. Para comenzar el tratamiento, tome 2 pastillas.
2. Luego, tome 1 pastilla después de cada evacuación con diarrea (cada vez que haga del dos).
3. No tome más de 8 pastillas al día.
4. Tome líquidos claros como caldos desgrasados o jugos.
   (Para niños: suero oral)

Efectos secundarios (molestias)
Este medicamento le puede provocar boca seca, somnolencia, cólicos, inflamación abdominal o estreñimiento.

Las preguntas fundamentales[2]
1. ¿Para qué es esta medicina?
2. ¿Cómo va a usar esta medicina?
3. ¿Cuáles son los efectos secundarios?
4. Me gustaría ver si le expliqué bien. Por favor, dígame cómo va a usar esta medicina.

Questions[3]

For an adult

1. How long have you had diarrhea?
2. How many times do you go to the bathroom each day?
3. Please describe the stools: Are they watery or liquid? Is there any blood or mucus?
4. Have you made any changes in your meals?
5. Have you traveled in the past few days? Did you travel abroad?
6. What medications or herbal remedies do you take? Are you taking an antibiotic?
7. Have you had other problems?
8. Do you have a fever?
9. Are you thirsty or feel that you have a dry mouth?
10. Do you have stomach upset, abdominal cramping, vomiting, or loss of appetite?
11. Have you had dizziness, confusion, irritability, or weakness?

For a child

How old is your son (daughter)?

1. How long has your child had diarrhea?
2. How many times has the child voided? How many times did he (she) go to the bathroom?
3. Please describe the child's stools: Are they watery or liquid? Is there any blood or mucus?
4. Did the child eat something different?
5. Has the child been to another house? Have you taken him (her) on a trip?
6. Have you given him (her) any medicine or herbal remedies? Are you giving him (her) any antibiotics?
7. Have you noticed any other symptoms besides the diarrhea?
8. Has the child had any fever?
9. Is the child thirsty or have you noticed that he (she) has a dry mouth?
10. Does the child complain of stomachache, abdominal cramping, or loss of appetite?
11. Have you noticed if the child has been dizzy, irritable, or very weak? Have you noticed if he (she) is confused?

Recommendations

Loperamide 2 mg (for an adult)

1. Take 2 pills to start.
2. Then, take 1 pill after each loose stool (diarrhea), each time you go to the bathroom (number 2).
3. Don't take more than 8 pills each day.
4. Take clear liquids like soups (without fat) or juices.
   (For children: oral rehydration liquids [Pedialyte®])

Side effects

This medication may cause dry mouth, drowsiness, abdominal cramping, bloating, or constipation.

Prime questions[2]

1. What is this medication for?
2. How are you going to use this medication?
3. What are the side effects?
4. I would like to see if I explained it well to you. Please tell me how you are going to use this medicine.

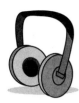

Diálogos para el audio

FARMACÉUTICA: Muy buenos días. Soy la Dra. Nguyen. ¿En qué le puedo ayudar?

PACIENTE: *Buenos días, doctora. Fíjese que mi hijo tiene diarrea. Ya lo llevé con el doctor de esta clínica. Me dijo que si mi hijo no se sentía mejor en un día le comprara un medicamento que se llama "lo-pra-mi" . . . o algo así.*

FARMACÉUTICA: Ah, muy bien. Pero antes quiero hacerle algunas preguntas. ¿Cuántos años tiene su hijo?

PACIENTE: *Acaba de cumplir 9 años.*

Preguntas[3]

1. ¿Desde cuándo ha tenido diarrea su hijo?
   Ha tenido diarrea desde hace 2 días.

2. ¿Cuántas veces al día va al baño?
   Va de cinco a seis veces al día, y lo veo que tiene que correr.

3. Por favor, describa los excrementos: ¿Son aguados o líquidos? ¿Hay sangre o moco?
   La popó es aguada y tiene poquito moco.

4. ¿Comió algo diferente?
   Pues, comimos con unos amigos en un restaurante nuevo durante el fin de semana.

5. ¿Ha ido a otra casa?
   No.

6. ¿Le está dando alguna medicina o algún remedio de hierbas? ¿Le está dando algún antibiótico?
   No, no le estoy dando nada.

7. ¿Le ha notado otros síntomas aparte de la soltura?
   Ahora no.

8. ¿Tiene fiebre?
   No, no tiene fiebre.

9. ¿Tiene sed o siente la boca reseca?
   Sí, últimamente he notado que toma mucha agua.

10. ¿Tiene dolor de estómago, cólicos, vómito o pérdida del apetito?
    Ha perdido un poco el apetito, pero creo que no tiene cólicos.

11. ¿Ha notado que esté mareado, irritable o muy débil?
    Sí, está muy irritable y también un poco débil.

Recomendaciones

Por ahora, déle muchos líquidos. Si todavía no se siente bien en un día, puede tomar la medicina como se la recomendó el doctor. La medicina se llama loperamide de 2 mg.

Para comenzar el tratamiento déle 1 pastilla tres veces al día, el primer día. Luego, déle 1 pastilla después de cada evacuación con soltura, pero no más de 3 pastillas al día. Después de 2 días, si todavía sigue la diarrea, consulte con su doctor otra vez. Déle mucha agua y líquidos claros como caldos desgrasados o jugos. También puede darle suero oral.

Efectos secundarios (molestias)

Este medicamento le puede provocar boca seca, somnolencia, cólicos, inflamación abdominal o estreñimiento.

Las preguntas fundamentales[2]

1. ¿Para qué es esta medicina?
   Es para la diarrea que tiene mi hijo.

2. ¿Cómo va a darle esta medicina?
   Para comenzar, voy a darle 1 pastilla tres veces al día en el primer día. Después voy a darle una cada vez que tenga diarrea, pero no más de 3 pastillas al día.

3. ¿Cuáles son los efectos secundarios?
   Puede provocarle somnolencia, cólicos, inflamación del abdomen, estreñimiento, o que se le reseque la boca.

4. Me gustaría ver si le expliqué bien. Por favor, dígame cómo va a darle esta medicina a su hijo.
   Voy a darle mucha agua, líquidos claros o suero oral por 1 día. Si todavía tiene diarrea, voy a darle 1 pastilla tres veces en el primer día. Después voy a darle 1 pastilla cada vez que tenga diarrea, pero no más de tres pastillas en un día. Puedo seguir dándole muchos líquidos. Después de 2 días, si sigue con diarrea, voy a llevarlo con el doctor otra vez.

Muy bien. Ojalá que su hijo se mejore pronto.

Muchas gracias, doctora.

Que le vaya bien.

◼ *Audio dialogues*

PHARMACIST: Good morning. I am Dr. Nguyen. How can I help you?

PATIENT: *Good morning, Doctor. You know, my son has diarrhea. I already took him to the doctor from this clinic. He told me that if my son doesn't feel better in a day, I should buy him a medication called "lo-pra-mi" . . . or something like that.*

PHARMACIST: Oh, very well. But first I want to ask you a few questions. How old is your son?

PATIENT: *He just turned (completed) 9 years.*

Questions[3]

1. How long has your son had diarrhea?
   He has had diarrhea for 2 days.

2. How many times does he go to the bathroom each day?
   He goes five to six times a day, and I see that he is running (to the bathroom).

3. Please describe the stools. Are they watery or liquid? Is there any blood or mucus?
   The stool is watery and has a little mucus.

4. Did he eat something different?
   Well, we ate with some friends at a new restaurant during the weekend.

5. Has he visited (gone to) another house?
   No.

6. Are you giving him any medication or an herbal remedy? Are you giving him an antibiotic?
   No, I am not giving him anything.

7. Have you noticed any other problems aside from the diarrhea?
   Not right now.

8. Does he have a fever?
   No, he doesn't have a fever.

9. Is he thirsty or does he have a dry mouth?
   Yes, I have noticed that he drinks a lot of water lately.

10. Does he have stomach upset, abdominal cramping, vomiting, or loss of appetite?
    He has lost his appetite a little, but I don't think he has had abdominal cramping.

11. Have you noticed that he has been dizzy, irritable, or very weak?
    Yes, he has been very irritable and also a little weak.

Recommendations

For now, give him a lot of liquids. If he still doesn't feel better in a day, he can take the medicine as recommended by the doctor. The medicine is called loperamide 2 mg.

To start the treatment, give him 1 pill three times a day for the first day. Then, give him 1 pill after each loose stool, but no more than 3 pills a day. After 2 days, if the diarrhea continues, consult with your doctor again. Give him a lot of water and clear liquids like soup (without fat) or juices. Also, you can give him oral rehydration drinks.

Side effects

This medication may cause dry mouth, drowsiness, abdominal cramping, bloating, or constipation.

Prime questions[2]

1. What is this medication for?
   It's for the diarrhea that my son has.

2. How are you going to give him this medication?
   To begin, I will give him 1 pill three times a day on the first day. Then, I will give him one pill each time that he has diarrhea but not more than 3 pills in a day.

3. What are the side effects?
   It can cause drowsiness, cramps, abdominal bloating, constipation, or dry mouth.

4. I would like to see if I explained it well to you. Please tell me how you are going to give this medicine to your son.
   I am going to give him lots of water, clear liquids, or oral rehydration drinks for 1 day. If he still has diarrhea, I will give him 1 pill three times on the first day. Then, I will give him 1 pill each time that he has diarrhea, but not more than three times in a day. I can continue to give him lots of liquids. After 2 days, if he continues with diarrhea, I will take him to the doctor again.

Very good! I hope that your son gets better soon.

Many thanks, Doctor.

May all go well.

De la cultura / About the culture

1. Common treatments for diarrhea in the Hispanic culture include drinking lots of beverages, mainly teas and "atoles" (a mixture of rice flour or cornstarch cooked in water with or without sugar). It is common to give infants rice flour instead of the usual milk formula (they don't drink milk when they have diarrhea). For adults, it is common to eat a diet of clear broths ("caldos") without fat or beverages without sugar.
2. Common treatments for constipation in some Hispanic cultures include a diet of prunes, lots of water, or a cup of warm water with lemon on an empty stomach. If the constipation is severe, people take purgatives or apply enemas.
3. In the English language, health care personnel often say that a drug "works" in the body. When translating to Spanish, "funcionar" is the more correct verb used to describe the way a drug functions in the body. The word "trabajar" most often refers to "work" as in an occupation.
4. The following vocabulary words can be used when talking about diarrhea and constipation. However, they are more technical or represent a higher level of vocabulary: "excrementos," "heces fecales," "estimular," "legumbres," and "obstrucción intestinal."
5. In some Hispanic cultures, patients will use the word "dieta" to refer to a diet that they are on to lose weight. They do not generally refer to diet as the regular foods that they eat. A word that can be used for regular foods is "alimentación" or "comida." Health care professionals often refer to "diet" as the normal foods that a person eats during a day.
6. In some Hispanic cultures, people can comfortably say "me duele el recto" to literally mean "my anus hurts." They will interchange the words for "anus" and "rectum." However, in U.S. culture, it is not as common to use these terms to describe pain during defecation.
7. When saying goodbye, many people will say "Que Dios lo bendiga," which means "God bless you." This expression is often acceptable, probably because of the high rate of Christianity in the population.

Apuntes de gramática / Grammar notes

Subjunctive: The subjunctive is verb mood that often follows a phrase expressing desires, hopes, or feelings. It often describes a state of possibility or probability as opposed to a certainty.

Example: Tómela a diario <u>para que</u> la medicina <u>funcione</u>.
Take it daily so that the medication works.

Ｌa doctora <u>quiere que</u> usted <u>tome</u> la medicina.
The doctor wants you to take the medicine.

Ejercicios / Exercises

I. Escriba una pregunta para cada respuesta. (Write a question for each answer.)

1. ¿_____?
   Lo mezclo con agua.

2. ¿_____?
   Viajamos a la playa.

3. ¿_____?
   Se pone una bolsita de té en una taza de agua caliente.

4. ¿_____?
   Los efectos secundarios pueden ser cólicos y diarrea.

II. Escriba una oración con las siguientes palabras. (Write a sentence using the following words.)

1. causar / inflamación abdominal

2. comer / fibra / comida

3. apetito / cambiar

4. medicina / estimular

III. Describa los siguientes términos. Use oraciones completas. (Describe the following terms. Use complete sentences.)

1. heces fecales _____

2. laxante _____

3. obstrucción intestinal _____

IV. Conjugue los verbos en subjuntivo. (Conjugate the verbs into subjunctive.)

La doctora quiere que . . .

1. (bajar de peso) _____.

2. (comer frutas y verduras) _____.

Yo recomiendo que usted . . .

3. (mezclar la medicina con agua) _____.

4. (tratar de tomar más agua) _____.

V. Busque en el Internet un sitio en español sobre uno de los temas siguientes. Escriba un párrafo sencillo para explicarle a un paciente. (Look up an Internet site in Spanish about one of the following topics. Write a simple paragraph to explain it to a patient.)

1. el estreñimiento

2. la diarrea

3. El cólera y la cólera (How does "la" or "el" change the meaning?)

REFERENCES

1. Curry CE Jr, Butler DM. Constipation. In: Berardi RR, Kroon LA, McDermott JH, et al., eds. *Handbook of Nonprescription Drugs.* 15th ed. Washington, DC: American Pharmacists Association; 2006:299–326.
2. Gardner M, Boyce RW, Herrier RN. *Pharmacist–Patient Consultation Program PPCP-Unit I: An Interactive Approach to Verifying Patient Understanding.* New York: Pfizer Educational Services; 1991.
3. Walker PC. Diarrhea. In: Berardi RR, Kroon LA, McDermott JH, et al., eds. *Handbook of Nonprescription Drugs.* 15th ed. Washington, DC: American Pharmacists Association; 2006:327–50.

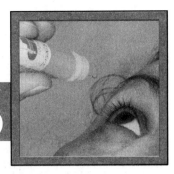

Capítulo
Chapter **5**

Productos oftálmicos y óticos
Eye and ear products

Verbos / Verbs

Presente / Present tense

Verbos / Verbs		Yo	Él, ella, usted	Mandato	Ejemplos
abrir(se)	to open	abro	abre	Abra	*Abra el ojo con los dedos.*
aplicar(se)	to apply, to instill	aplico	aplica	Aplique	*Aplíquese la pomada.*
arder	to sting	me arde	le arde	—	*Me arden los ojos.*
calentar	to heat, to warm	caliento	calienta	Caliente	*No caliente las gotas.*
cerrar	to close	cierro	cierra	Cierre	*Cierre bien la medicina.*
deber (de)	should, must	debo (de)	debe (de)	—	*Debe (de) ponerle la pomada.*
dejar	to permit, to allow	dejo	deja	Deje	*No deje que se mueva.*
despertar(se)	to wake up	(me) despierto	(se) despierta	Despiértese	*No despierte al niño.*
escuchar	to listen	escucho	escucha	Escuche	*Escuche a su doctor.*
inclinar(se)	to tilt, to lean	inclino	inclina	Incline	*Incline la cabeza hacia atrás.*
jalar(se)	to pull	jalo	jala	Jale	*Jálele la oreja hacia arriba.*
lavar(se)	to wash	lavo	lava	Lave	*Lávese con agua y jabón.*
limpiar(se)	to clean	limpio	limpia	Limpie	*Limpie el exceso con un algodón.*
mantener(se)	to keep, to stay	mantengo	mantiene	Mantenga	*Mantenga las medicinas fuera del alcance de los niños.*
mirar	to look	miro	mira	Mire	*Mire hacia arriba.*
mover(se)	to move	(me) muevo	(se) mueve	Muévase	*No se mueva, por favor.*
oir	to hear	oigo	oye	Oiga	*Oigo zumbidos.*
oprimir(se)	to press	oprimo	oprime	Oprima	*Oprímase ligeramente el lagrimal con el dedo.*

continued on p. 80

Verbos / Verbs		Presente / Present tense			
		Yo	Él, ella, usted	Mandato	Ejemplos
parpadear	to blink	parpadeo	parpadea	Parpadee	*Parpadee suavemente.*
permanecer	to keep, to stay	permanezco	permanece	Permanezca	*Permanezca unos momentos con los ojos cerrados.*
poner(se)	to place, to put	pongo	pone	Ponga	*Póngase una a dos gotas en cada oído.*
refrigerar	to refrigerate	refrigero	refrigera	Refrigere	*No refrigere las gotas.*
seguir	to follow	sigo	sigue	Siga	*Siga las instrucciones al pie de la letra.*
soltar	to release	suelto	suelta	Suelte	*Suelte el párpado después de aplicar las gotas.*
supurar	to suppurate (pus), to ooze	me supura me supuran	le supura le supuran	—	*¿Le supura el ojo?*
tocar	to touch	toco	toca	Toque	*No se toque el ojo con el tubo de la pomada.*
ver	to see	veo	ve	Vea	*Vea a su médico.*

Las partes de los ojos y los oídos /Parts of the eyes and ears

la ceja	eyebrow
el iris	iris
el lagrimal	tear duct
"la lengüeta" de la oreja	tragus, "earflap"
el lóbulo de la oreja	ear lobe
el oído	inner ear
el ojo	eye
la oreja	outer ear
el párpado	eyelid
la pestaña	eyelash
la pupila	pupil
el tímpano	eardrum

Sustantivos / Nouns

la cerilla, el cerumen	earwax
el frasco	vial, small bottle
la gota	drop
el hormigueo	tingling (like ants)
el jabón	soap
las lagañas	"sleep" in the eye
los lentes, los anteojos, las gafas	eyeglasses
el oftalmólogo	ophthalmologist
el orificio	orifice, opening
la pomada	ointment
la punzada	sharp pain

el segundo	second
el sobrante	excess

Adjetivos / Adjectives

borroso(a)	blurry
ciego(a)	blind
claro(a)	clear
infectado(a)	infected
intenso(a)	intense
irritado(a)	irritated
pequeño(a)	little
sordo(a)	mute

Otras expresiones / Other expressions

a fondo	thoroughly
demasiado	too much
de tal manera	in such a way
directamente	directly
en ocasiones	at times
estar(se) quieto	to stay still
hacia	toward
por lo menos	at least
por un rato	for a while
suavemente	smoothly
temporalmente	temporarily

Direcciones / Directions

abajo	down, below
adentro	inside
alrededor	around
antes	before
arriba	up, above

debajo	underneath, below
(a la) derecha	to the right
derecho	straight, straight ahead
(a la) izquierda	to the left

Problemas de los ojos / Eye conditions

la(s) alergia(s)	allergy(ies)
la ceguera	blindness
la conjuntivitis	conjunctivitis
el glaucoma	glaucoma
la(s) infección(es)	infection(s)
los ojos resecos	dry eyes
los ojos rojos	red eyes (slang)
el orzuelo, la perrilla	stye
la visión borrosa	blurry vision

Problemas de los oídos / Ear conditions

el dolor de oído	earache
la infección	infection
el (la) mudo(a)	mute
el oído de nadador	swimmer's ear
la otitis media	otitis media
la punzada de oído	earache
la sordera	deafness
la supuración	suppuration
el tinnitus	tinnitus (ringing)
el vértigo	vertigo
el zumbido	ringing

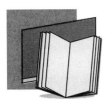

Lección 1 Gotas para los ojos
Lesson 1 Eye drops

Note: This lesson uses the reflexive pronoun ("se") with some verbs to describe how patients should apply medication to themselves.

Preguntas[1]

1. ¿Le duelen los ojos? ¿Le arden los ojos?
2. ¿Tiene comezón en los ojos? ¿Tiene los ojos rojos? ¿Le pican?
3. ¿Le lloran los ojos? ¿Le supuran?
4. ¿Tiene visión borrosa?
5. ¿Usa lentes (anteojos, gafas) o lentes de contacto?
6. ¿Desde cuándo le molestan los ojos?
7. ¿Qué hizo para aliviar el problema?

Recomendación

Esta medicina es para los ojos resecos (o infectados).
Póngase (Aplíquese) de 1 a 2 gotas . . .

   . . . en cada ojo
   . . . en ambos ojos
   . . . en el ojo derecho
   . . . en el ojo izquierdo
   . . . en el ojo afectado
     . . . dos veces al día mientras esté despierto.

Instrucciones

1. Lávese las manos con agua y jabón.
2. Incline la cabeza hacia atrás.
3. Ábrase el ojo con los dedos (así).
4. Antes de aplicar la primera gota, mire hacia arriba.
5. Aplíquese las gotas.
6. Cierre los ojos y espere de 1 a 2 minutos.
7. No parpadee.
8. Apriétese el lagrimal con un dedo.

Efectos secundarios (molestias)

Puede causar visión borrosa.

Recomendaciones adicionales

1. Si no siente la solución, refrigérela antes de aplicarla.
2. Si necesita más de 1 gota, espere por lo menos 5 minutos entre cada aplicación adicional.
3. Si tiene que aplicar pomada también, aplíquese las gotas por lo menos 10 minutos antes que la pomada.

Las preguntas fundamentales[2]

1. ¿Para qué es esta medicina?
2. ¿Cómo va a aplicarse esta medicina?
3. ¿Cuáles son los efectos secundarios?
4. Me gustaría confirmar la información. Por favor, dígame cómo va a usar esta medicina.

Questions[1]

1. Do your eyes hurt? Do they sting you?
2. Are your eyes itchy? Are they red? Do they burn?
3. Are your eyes weeping? Do they have pus?
4. Do you have blurry vision?
5. Do you use eyeglasses or contact lenses?
6. How long have your eyes bothered you?
7. What have you done to alleviate the problem?

Recommendation

This medicine is for dry (or infected) eyes.
Put (yourself) 1 to 2 drops in . . .

     . . . each eye
     . . . both eyes
     . . . the right eye
     . . . the left eye
     . . . the affected eye
          . . . twice a day while you are awake.

Instructions

1. Wash your hands with water and soap.
2. Lean your head back.
3. Open your eye with your fingers (like this).
4. Before applying the first drop, look up.
5. Instill the drop (to yourself).
6. Close your eyes and wait for 1 to 2 minutes.
7. Don't blink.
8. Squeeze (press) your tear duct with a finger.

Side effects

It may cause blurry vision.

Additional recommendations

1. If you don't feel the solution, refrigerate it before applying it.
2. If you need more than 1 drop, wait for at least 5 minutes between each additional application.
3. If you have to apply an ointment also, instill the drops (to yourself) at least 10 minutes before the ointment.

Prime questions[2]

1. What is this medication for?
2. How are you going to use this medication?
3. What are the side effects?
4. I would like to confirm the information. Please tell me how you are going to use this medicine.

Diálogos para el audio

FARMACÉUTICA: Buenos días. Me llamo Cynthia Flores. Soy la farmacéutica y hablo inglés y español. ¿Lo puedo ayudar en algo?

PACIENTE: *Ay, señorita, muy buenos días. Soy José Raúl Leal. ¡Qué bueno que usted habla español! Sabe que los ojos me molestan mucho. Los traigo muy irritados. No soy de aquí. Estoy de viaje y no hablo inglés muy bien.*

FARMACÉUTICA: Entiendo. Debo hacerle algunas preguntas antes de recomendarle algún producto para aliviar las molestias.

Preguntas[1]

1. ¿Le duelen los ojos? ¿Le arden los ojos?
   No, no me duelen los ojos, pero sí los siento irritados.

2. ¿Tiene comezón en los ojos? ¿Tiene los ojos rojos? ¿Le pican?
   Sí, tengo comezón en los ojos y me pican—es decir, me arden mucho. A veces están rojos, creo que de tanto tallármelos.

3. ¿Le lloran los ojos? ¿Tiene lagañas? ¿Le supuran?
   No, al contrario, no me lloran, están resecos. Siento como si trajera arena en los ojos.

4. ¿Tiene visión borrosa?
   No, no he tenido visión borrosa, pero no veo como antes.

5. ¿Usa lentes o lentes de contacto?
   Uso lentes de contacto. Los he usado desde hace 2 años y nunca había tenido ningún problema.

6. ¿Desde cuándo le molestan los ojos?
   Me han molestado los ojos desde hace una semana con el cambio de clima y tanto polvo.

7. ¿Qué ha hecho para tratar de aliviar el problema?
   Bueno, me quité los lentes de contacto y ahora estoy usando mis gafas pero no veo igual. Prefiero usar mis lentes de contacto, pero cuando me los puse hoy por la mañana no los aguanté y me los quité. ¿Hay algo que me pueda recomendar?

Recomendación

Bueno, estas gotas son para los ojos resecos y enrojecidos. Póngase de 1 a 2 gotas en ambos ojos tres o cuatro veces al día si es necesario.

¡Ah, muy bien, Srta. Flores! Pero nunca he usado gotas para los ojos.

Instrucciones

Para usarlas . . .
1. Lávese las manos con agua y jabón.
2. Incline la cabeza hacia atrás.
3. Ábrase el ojo con los dedos (así).
4. Antes de aplicar la primera gota, mire hacia arriba.
5. Aplíquese las gotas.
6. Cierre los ojos y espere de 1 a 2 minutos.
7. No parpadee.
8. Apriétese suavemente el lagrimal con un dedo.

Efectos secundarios (molestias)

Estas gotas pueden causarle visión borrosa por un rato.

Recomendaciones adicionales

1. Si no siente la solución, refrigérela antes de aplicarla.
2. Si hay alguna razón para usar otros productos para los ojos, espere por lo menos 5 minutos entre cada aplicación adicional.
3. Si tiene que aplicarse una pomada también, aplíquese las gotas por lo menos 10 minutos antes que la pomada.

Las preguntas fundamentales[2]

1. ¿Para qué es esta medicina?
   Esta medicina es para los ojos resecos y enrojecidos.

2. ¿Cómo va a aplicarse esta medicina?
   Me voy a poner de 1 a 2 gotas en ambos ojos hasta cuatro veces al día si es necesario.

3. ¿Cuáles son los efectos secundarios?
   Puede causarme visión borrosa.

4. Me gustaría confirmar la información. Por favor, dígame cómo va a usar esta medicina.
   Sí, claro. Esta medicina es para los ojos resecos y enrojecidos. Me voy a poner de 1 a 2 gotas en ambos ojos hasta cuatro veces al día si es necesario. Puede causarme visión borrosa.

Muy bien, Sr. Leal. También, lave bien los lentes de contacto. Revise que sus lentes no tengan ninguna abrasión. Espere 15 minutos después de usar el medicamento para volver a ponerse los lentes de contacto. Si no siente alivio dentro de una semana o si las molestias empeoran, es recomendable consultar con un médico u oftalmólogo inmediatamente. Que se sienta mejor.

Muchas gracias, muy amable.

Audio dialogues

PHARMACIST: Good morning. My name is Cynthia Flores. I am the pharmacist, and I speak English and Spanish. How can I help you with something?

PATIENT: *Yes, Miss, very good morning. I am José Raúl Leal. I'm so glad that you speak Spanish! You see my eyes are bothering me. They are (I "carry them") very irritated. I'm not from here. I am traveling (on a trip) and I do not speak English very well.*

PHARMACIST: I understand. I will need to ask you some questions before recommending (to you) a product to alleviate the discomfort.

Questions[1]

1. Do your eyes hurt? Do they burn?
   No, my eyes don't really hurt me, but they are irritated.

2. Are your eyes itchy? Are they red? Do they sting you?
   Yes, they itch and they sting me—that is to say, they burn (me) a lot. Sometimes, they are red, I think because I rub them so much.

3. Do your eyes tear? Are your eyes weepy? Do they have pus?
   No, on the contrary, my eyes do not tear—they are dry. I feel like my eyes have sand in them.

4. Do you have blurry vision?
   No, I haven't had blurry vision, but I don't see as well as before.

5. Do you use eyeglasses or contact lenses?
   I use contact lenses. I have used them for 2 years, and I've never had any problems.

6. How long have your eyes bothered you?
   My eyes have bothered me since last week with the change in weather and all of the dust.

7. What have you done to try to alleviate the problem?
   Well, I took out my contact lenses and now I am using my glasses, but I do not see the same. I prefer to use my contact lenses, but when I put them on this morning I could not bear them and I took them out. Is there something that you can recommend for me?

Recommendation

Well, this medicine is to treat dry and red eyes.
Place 1 to 2 drops in both (of your) eyes three or four times a day if necessary.

Oh, very good, Miss Flores. But I have never used eye drops.

Instructions

To use them . . .
1. Wash your hands with water and soap.
2. Lean your head back.
3. Open your eye with your fingers (like this).
4. Before applying the first drop, look up.
5. Instill the drops (yourself).
6. Close your eyes and wait for 1 to 2 minutes.
7. Don't blink.
8. Squeeze (press) your tear duct gently with a finger.

Side effects

These drops may cause you to have blurry vision for a while.

Additional recommendations

1. If you don't feel the solution, refrigerate it before applying it.
2. If there is some reason to use another eye product, wait for at least 5 minutes between each additional application.
3. If you also have to apply (yourself) an ointment, instill the drops at least 10 minutes before the ointment.

Prime questions[2]

1. What is this medication for?
   This medicine is for dry and reddened eyes.

2. How are you going to use this medication?
   I am going to put (myself) 1 to 2 drops in both eyes up to four times a day if necessary.

3. What are the side effects?
   It can cause (me) blurry vision.

4. I would like to confirm the information. Please tell me how you are going to use this medicine.
   Yes, of course. This medicine is for dry and reddened eyes. I am going to put (myself) 1 to 2 drops in both eyes up to four times a day if necessary. It may cause (me) blurry vision.

Very well, Mr. Leal. Also, wash your contact lenses well. Check that your lenses don't have any scratches. Wait 15 minutes after you use the medication before you put your contact lenses in.
If you don't get better or the symptoms worsen, it's recommended that you see your doctor or ophthalmologist immediately. I hope you feel better.

Thank you very much, (you are) very kind.

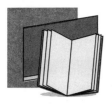

Lección 2   Pomada para los ojos
Lesson 2   Eye ointment

Note: In this lesson, the authors have included the reflexive ("se") and indirect object pronouns ("le, se"). This inclusion should help bring up discussion about how to tell patients to apply medication to themselves or to another person (e.g., a child).

Las preguntas fundamentales para medicamentos recetados[2]*

1. ¿Para qué le dijo el doctor (la doctora) que era esta medicina?
2. ¿Cómo le dijo el doctor (la doctora) que se pusiera esta medicina?
3. ¿Qué le dijo el doctor (la doctora) que le podía pasar con esta medicina?

Recomendación[3]

Ejemplo: Eritromicina al 0.5% en pomada para una infección de los ojos

Apliquese(le)† una cantidad muy pequeña de la medicina en el párpado de abajo . . .

   . . . de cada ojo
   . . . de ambos ojos
   . . . del ojo derecho
   . . . del ojo izquierdo
   . . . del ojo afectado
      . . . de ____ a ____ veces al día mientras esté despierto(a).

Instrucciones[1]

1. Debe lavarse bien las manos con agua y jabón.
2. Incline(le) la cabeza hacia atrás.
3. Ábrase(le) con cuidado el ojo con los dedos (así).
4. Apriete el tubo para aplicarse(le) la pomada dentro del párpado (del niño o de la niña). No se (le) toque el ojo con la punta del tubo.
5. Cierre (Haga que el niño o la niña cierre) los ojos suavemente de 1 a 2 minutos.

Efectos secundarios (molestias)

Puede causarle visión borrosa o una molestia ligera en los ojos.

Recomendaciones adicionales

Si necesita ponerse(le) gotas también, apliquese(le) las gotas por lo menos 10 minutos antes de la pomada.

Las preguntas fundamentales[2]

1. ¿Para qué es esta medicina?
2. ¿Cómo se (le) va a poner esta medicina (en los ojos de su hijo o hija)?
3. ¿Cuáles son los efectos secundarios?
4. Quiero estar seguro(a) que no olvidé nada. Por favor, dígame cómo va a usar esta medicina.

---

*This is the first time the text refers to a prescription medication. The prime questions include queries about the doctor's explanation of the medication.
†The pronoun "se" is used when the person is talking about him/herself. The pronoun "le" is used when talking about applying to someone else.

Prime questions for prescription medication[2]
What did the doctor tell you the medicine was for?
How did the doctor tell you to apply the medicine?
What did the doctor tell you to expect (that could happen to you) from this medicine?

Recommendation
Example: Erythromycin ointment 0.5% for an eye infection[3]

Apply to yourself (to him or her) a small amount of medication in the lower eyelid . . .

    . . . of each eye
    . . . of both eyes
    . . . of the right eye
    . . . of the left eye
    . . . of the affected eye
        . . . from _____ to _____ times a day while awake.

Directions[1]
1. You should wash your hands well with water and soap.
2. Lean your (his or her) head back.
3. Open your (his or her) eyes carefully with the fingers (like this).
4. Squeeze the tube to apply to yourself (him or her) the ointment inside the eyelid (of the child). Do not touch your (his or her) eye with the tip of the tube.
5. Close your (Have the child close his or her) eyes gently for 1 to 2 minutes.

Side effects
It may cause you (him or her) blurry vision or slight eye discomfort.

Additional recommendations
If you (he or she) also need to apply eye drops, apply to yourself (him or her) the drops at least 10 minutes before the ointment.

Prime questions[2]
1. What is this medication for?
2. How are you going to apply to yourself (him or her) this medication (in your son's or daughter's eyes)?
3. What are the side effects?
4. I want to be sure that I didn't forget anything. Please tell me how you are going to use this medicine.

Diálogos para el audio

FARMACÉUTICO: Buenas noches. Me llamo Richard Stevens y soy el farmacéutico. ¿Cómo le puedo ayudar?

PACIENTE: *Buenas noches, Sr. Stevens. Pues, mi hijo ha traído el ojo izquierdo muy rojo desde el lunes. También tiene comezón, irritación e inflamación alrededor del ojo. Por las mañanas amanece con lagañas en el párpado y se rasca mucho. Temo que se le pase al otro ojo. Hoy en la mañana la maestra me dijo que el niño no podía asistir a la escuela hasta que se aliviara. El doctor lo checó ayer. Aquí traigo la receta.*

FARMACÉUTICO: Gracias, ahora se la preparo.

PACIENTE: *Aquí lo espero, señor, gracias.*

[una pausa]

Pues, aquí tiene la medicina. Pero me gustaría hacerle algunas preguntas.

Las preguntas fundamentales para medicamentos recetados[2]

1. ¿Para qué le dijo el doctor que era esta medicina?
   Bueno, para la infección de los ojos de mi hijo.

2. ¿Cómo le dijo el doctor que le pusiera esta medicina?
   No me ha dicho. ¿Me puede explicar cómo aplicarla?

3. ¿Qué le dijo el doctor que le podía pasar con esta medicina?
   Tampoco me dijo nada.

Recomendación[3]

1. Bueno, el doctor le recetó a su hijo una pomada de eritromicina para tratar la conjuntivitis, una infección de ojos. Es contagiosa pero no es grave. Debe empezar a aplicársela hoy mismo.
2. Aplíquele a su hijo la medicina en el párpado de abajo del ojo izquierdo tres veces al día, mientras esté despierto.
3. Le voy a dar algunas instrucciones adicionales.

Instrucciones[1]

1. Debe lavarse bien las manos con agua y jabón antes y después de aplicarle el medicamento a su hijo.
2. Inclínele la cabeza hacia atrás.
3. Ábrale con cuidado el ojo izquierdo con los dedos, así.
4. Apriete el tubo para aplicarle una cantidad pequeña de la pomada dentro del párpado del niño. No le toque el ojo con la punta del tubo.
5. Haga que el niño cierre los ojos suavemente de 1 a 2 minutos.

Efectos secundarios (molestias)

La pomada puede causarle visión borrosa o una molestia muy ligera en los ojos.

Recomendaciones adicionales

1. Si necesita ponerle gotas también, aplíquele las gotas por lo menos 10 minutos antes de la pomada.
2. Para evitar el contagio al ojo derecho o a otros miembros de la familia, el niño debe evitar tocarse los ojos con las manos. Toda la familia debe lavarse las manos con frecuencia.
3. Si los síntomas persisten más de 3 o 4 días, debe consultar con su médico otra vez.

Las preguntas fundamentales[2]

Entonces, por favor explíqueme . . .

1. ¿Cómo va a ponerle la pomada a su hijo?
   Antes de aplicarle el medicamento voy a lavarme las manos muy bien con agua y jabón. Voy a inclinarle la cabeza hacia atrás. Tengo que abrirle con cuidado el ojo afectado con mis dedos y aplicarle la pomada tres veces al día. No debo tocarle el párpado con la punta del tubo. El niño debe permanecer con los ojos cerrados suavemente unos 2 minutos después de ponerle la pomada.

2. ¿Cuáles son los efectos secundarios?
   Puede causarle visión borrosa o una molestia muy ligera en los ojos.

3. Quiero estar seguro que no olvidé nada. Por favor, dígame cómo va a usar esta medicina.
   Sí, claro. Voy a aplicarle a mi hijo una pequeña cantidad de pomada en el ojo izquierdo tres veces al día. También, nos debemos lavar muy bien las manos con frecuencia.

Está bien. Pues, ojalá que su hijo se mejore.

Gracias, Sr. Stevens.

Audio dialogues

PHARMACIST: Good evening. My name is Richard Stevens, and I am the pharmacist. How may I help you?

PATIENT: *Good evening, Mr. Stevens. Well, my son's left eye has been quite red since Monday. He also has itching, irritation, and inflammation around his eye. In the mornings, he wakes up with "sleep" in his eyelid, and he scratches his eye frequently. I'm afraid that it will pass to his other eye. Today, in the morning, his teacher told me that he could not attend school until he was better. The doctor checked him yesterday. Here, I have brought you the prescription.*

PHARMACIST: Thank you. I'll get the prescription ready for you.

PATIENT: *I will wait here for you, sir. Thank you.*

[pause]

Well, here is the medicine. But I would like to ask you a few questions.

Prime questions for prescription medications[2]

1. What did the doctor tell you this medicine was for?
   Well, for the infection of the eyes of my son.

2. How did the doctor tell you to apply this medicine (to him)?
   He didn't tell me. Can you explain to me how to apply it?

3. What did the doctor tell you to expect (that could happen to him) from this medicine?
   (Neither) he told me nothing.

Recommendation[3]

1. Well, the doctor has prescribed your son an erythromycin ointment to treat conjunctivitis, an eye infection. It is contagious but is not serious. You should start applying it to him today.
2. Apply the medicine to your son in the lower eyelid of his left eye three times a day, while he is awake.
3. I am going to give you some additional directions.

Directions[1]

1. You should wash your hands well with water and soap before and after applying the medication to your son.
2. Lean his head toward the back.
3. Open carefully his left eye with your fingers, like this.
4. Squeeze the tube to apply a small amount of the ointment inside your son's eyelid. Do not touch his eye with the tip of the tube.
5. Have him close his eyes gently for 1 to 2 minutes.

Side effects

The ointment may cause him blurry vision or slight discomfort in the eyes.

Additional recommendations

1. If you also need to put eye drops in him, apply the drops in him at least 10 minutes before the ointment.
2. To avoid contamination of the right eye or of other family members, the boy should avoid touching his eyes with his hands. The whole family should wash their hands frequently.
3. If the symptoms persist more than 3 or 4 days, you should contact your doctor again.

Prime questions[2]

1. What is this medication for?
   It is a treatment for conjunctivitis.

2. How are you going to apply the ointment to your son?
   Before applying the medication to him, I am going to wash my hands very well with water and soap. I am going to tilt his head backward. I have to open carefully his affected eye with my fingers and apply the ointment to him three times a day. I should not touch his eyelid with the tip of the tube. My son should keep his eyes closed gently for some 2 minutes after I apply the ointment to him.

3. What are the side effects?
   It may cause him blurry vision or a slight eye discomfort.

4. I want to be sure that I didn't forget anything. Please tell me how you are going to use this medicine.
   Yes, of course. I am going to apply to my son a small amount of ointment in the left eye three times a day. Also, we should wash our hands very well and frequently.

That's good. Well, I hope that your son gets better.

Thank you, Mr. Stevens.

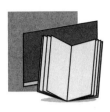

Lección 3 Gotas para los oídos
Lesson 3 Ear drops

Preguntas[4]

1. ¿Le duelen los oídos?
2. ¿Oye ruidos? ¿Tiene zumbidos en el oído?
3. ¿Ha tenido problemas para oír últimamente?
4. ¿En estos últimos días, ha ido a nadar?
5. ¿Se ha resfriado últimamente?

Recomendación[3]

Ejemplo: Cortisporin® en solución para el oído de nadador

Póngase de _____ a _____ gotas en . . .
>. . . cada oído
>. . . ambos oídos
>. . . el oído derecho
>. . . el oído izquierdo
>. . . el oído afectado
>>. . . de _____ a _____ veces al día.

Instrucciones

1. Lávese bien las manos con agua y jabón.
2. Límpiese(le) la oreja.
3. No caliente las gotas.
4. Agite el frasco (si es necesario).
5. Incline(le) la cabeza hacia el lado (derecho o izquierdo).
6. No se (le) toque la oreja con la punta del gotero.
7. Jálese(le) suavemente la oreja hacia atrás y hacia arriba. *Nota*: Si el paciente es un niño menor de 3 años, jálele con cuidado la oreja hacia atrás y hacia abajo.
8. Aplíquese(le) las gotas. (Aplíqueselas.)
9. Oprímase(le) la lengüeta de la oreja después de aplicarse(le) las gotas.
10. No se mueva por un ratito.
11. Si es un niño(a), póngale un algodón en el oído después de aplicarle las gotas.

Efectos secundarios (molestias)

Puede sentir un ligero hormigueo en los oídos.

Las preguntas fundamentales[2]

1. ¿Para qué es esta medicina?
2. ¿Cómo va a aplicar esta medicina?
3. ¿Cuáles son los efectos secundarios?
4. Quiero estar seguro(a) de que no olvidé nada. Por favor, dígame cómo va a usar esta medicina.

Questions[4]

1. Do your ears hurt?
2. Do you hear noises? Do you have ringing in your ears?
3. Have you had problems hearing lately?
4. In the past few days, have you gone swimming?
5. Have you had a cold lately?

Recommendation[3]

Example: Cortisporin® solution for swimmer's ear

Put from _____ to _____ drops in . . .

    . . . each ear

    . . . both ears

    . . . the right ear

    . . . the left ear

    . . . the affected ear

        . . . from ____ to ____ times a day.

Directions

1. Wash your hands well with water and soap.
2. Clean your (his or her) (outer) ears.
3. Don't heat the ear drops.
4. Shake the bottle (if needed).
5. Lean your (his or her) head to the (right or left) side.
6. Don't touch your (his or her) ear with the tip of the dropper.
7. Pull your (his or her) ear gently toward the back and up. *Note:* If the patient is a child under 3 years of age, pull his or her ear carefully to the back and down.
8. Put the drops in your (his or her) ears. (Put them in his or her ears.)
9. Press your (his or her) "earflap" after applying the drops.
10. Don't move (yourself) for a short time.
11. If the patient is a child, put a cotton ball in his ear after applying the drops to him.

Side effects

You may feel a slight tingling sensation (like ants) in your ears.

Prime questions[2]

1. What is this medication for?
2. How are you going to apply this medication?
3. What are the side effects?
4. I want to be sure that I didn't forget anything. Please tell me how you are going to use this medicine.

Diálogos para el audio

PACIENTE: *Hola, señorita, necesito ayuda. Me llamo Cecilia Sáenz. ¿Usted me podría surtir una receta para mi hija Julie?*

FARMACÉUTICA: Claro. Yo soy la farmacéutica, la Dra. Olimpia Andrews. ¿Cuál es el problema?

PACIENTE: *Mi hija se queja de punzadas en los oídos. Esta mañana la llevé con el doctor y aquí, traigo la receta.*

FARMACÉUTICA: Entiendo. ¿Qué edad tiene su hija?

PACIENTE: *Julie tiene casi 6 años.*

Preguntas[4]

1. ¿Le duelen los oídos a su hija?
   Sí, le duelen y le molestan los oídos. Bueno, se queja de que el oído derecho le molesta más.

2. ¿Oye ruidos? ¿Tiene zumbidos en los oídos?
   No, no creo que ella tenga zumbidos en los oídos.

3. ¿Ha tenido problemas para oír últimamente? ¿Oye bien?
   Ella no ha perdido el oído últimamente. Oye muy bien, bueno, ¡cuando quiere!

4. ¿Ha ido a nadar recientemente?
   Sí, fue a nadar hace 2 días. Se reunieron 15 niñas en la piscina de una amiga. Estuvieron en la piscina casi todo el día.

5. ¿Se ha resfriado recientemente?
   No, no se ha resfriado.

Recomendación

Pues, esta receta es para el oído de nadador que es una infección muy común en los niños. La medicina es una solución de Cortisporin®. Aplíquele 3 gotas en ambos oídos cuatro veces al día.

Instrucciones

1. Primero, lávese bien las manos con agua y jabón antes y después de aplicarle las gotas.
2. Límpiele las orejas.
3. No caliente las gotas.
4. Agite el frasco ligeramente.
5. Inclínele la cabeza hacia el lado izquierdo, y después de aplicarle las gotas, hacia el lado derecho.
6. No le toque la oreja con la punta del gotero.
7. Jálele suavemente la oreja hacia atrás y hacia arriba.
8. Aplíquele las gotas.
9. Oprímale la lengüeta de la oreja después de aplicarle las gotas.
10. No deje que se mueva por un ratito.
11. Puede ponerle un algodón en los oídos después de aplicarle las gotas.

Efectos secundarios (molestias)

Es posible que sienta un ligero hormigueo al aplicarle las gotas. Pero por lo general, no tiene molestias fuertes.

Las preguntas fundamentales[2]

Le di muchas instrucciones. Entonces, quiero confirmar que le expliqué bien.

1. ¿Para qué es esta medicina?
   Es para los oídos.

2. ¿Cómo va a aplicar esta medicina?
   Primero, me tengo que lavar bien las manos. Le limpio las orejas. Luego, le tengo que inclinar la cabeza hacia los lados para ponerle las gotas. Le jalo la oreja hacia atrás y hacia arriba. Puedo ponerle un algodón en los oídos. Le tengo que poner las gotas cuatro veces al día.

3. ¿Cuáles son los efectos secundarios?
   Pues, creo que no los hay.

4. Quiero estar segura de que no olvidé nada. Por favor, dígame cómo va a aplicarle esta medicina.
   Sí, claro. Voy a ponerle 3 gotas en los dos oídos cuatro veces al día.

Bueno, creo que entendió muy bien. Ojalá que su hija se mejore.

Muchas gracias, doctora.

■ *Audio dialogues*

PATIENT: *Hello, miss, I need some help. My name is Cecilia Saenz. Can you help me fill a prescription for my daughter Julie?*

PHARMACIST: Sure. I am the pharmacist, Dr. Olimpia Andrews. What is the problem?

PATIENT: *My daughter complains of sharp pain in her ears. This morning I took her to the doctor, and here, I have brought you a prescription.*

PHARMACIST: I understand. How old is your daughter?

PATIENT: *Julie is almost 6 years old.*

Questions[4]

1. Do your child's ears hurt?
   Yes, her ears hurt and they bother her. Well, she complains that the right ear bothers her more.

2. Does she hear noises? Does she have ringing in her ears?
   No, I don't think that she has ringing in her ears.

3. Has she had problems hearing lately? Does she hear well?
   She has not had any hearing loss lately. She hears very well, when she wants to!

4. Has she gone swimming recently?
   Yes, she went swimming 2 days ago. Fifteen girls got together at a friend's swimming pool. They were in the pool almost all day.

5. Has she had a cold recently?
   No, she has not had a cold.

Recommendation

Well, this prescription is for swimmer's ear, an infection very common in children. The medicine is a Cortisporin® solution. Instill 3 drops in both of her ears four times a day.

Directions

1. First, wash your hands well with water and soap, before and after applying the ear drops to her.
2. Clean her (outer) ears.
3. Don't heat the ear drops.
4. Shake the bottle slightly.
5. Lean her head toward the left side, and after applying the drops to her, toward the right side.
6. Don't touch her ear with the dropper tip.
7. Pull her ear gently toward the back and up.
8. Apply the drops to her (ear).
9. Press her "earflap" after applying the drops.
10. Don't allow her to move for a short time.
11. You can put a cotton ball in her ears after applying the drops (to her ears).

Side effects

It is possible that she may feel a slight tingling sensation (like ants) when you apply the drops (to her ears). But for the most part, it does not have strong side effects.

Prime questions[2]

I gave you a lot of instructions. So I would like to confirm that I explained (it) to you well.

1. What is this medication for?
   It is for the ears.

2. How are you going to apply this medication?
   First, I have to wash my hands well. I will clean her ears. Then, I have to lean her head toward the sides to put in the drops (in her ears). I pull her (outer) ear toward the back and up. I can put a piece of cotton in her ears. I have to put the drops (in her ears) four times a day.

3. What are the side effects?
   Well, I don't think there are any.

4. I want to be sure that I didn't forget anything. Please tell me how you are going to use this medicine.
   Yes, of course. I will put 3 drops in both her ears four times a day.

Good, I think you understood very well. I hope that your daughter gets better.

Many thanks, Doctor.

De la cultura / About the culture

1. Here are some ways that patients from Mexico may complain about an eye problem:

   "Tengo muchas lagañas."
   > (I have a lot of "sleep" in my eyes.)

   "Por la mañana amanezco con los ojos pegados."
   > (In the morning, I wake up with my eyes stuck together.)

   "Me lloran mucho los ojos y los tengo rojos."
   > (My eyes "weep" a lot, and they are red.)

2. Here are some ways that patients from Mexico may complain about an ear problem:

   "Tengo punzadas muy fuertes en este oído."
   > (I have a sharp pain in this ear.)

   "Me supura el oído y lo tengo muy caliente todo el tiempo."
   > (My ear "oozes," and I feel warm all of the time.)

   "Tengo un zumbido en este oído."
   > (I have a ringing in this ear.)

3. In Latin America, it is very common to use an eyewash ("lavaojos") with chamomile for an infection or for tired eyes.

4. The verbs "mover(se)" and "mudar(se)" can both be translated in English to "to move (oneself)." However, "mover(se)" generally refers to moving an object or a part of the body. "Mudar(se)" or "cambiar(se)" generally refers to location (e.g., to move from one city to another). However, along some parts of the United States–Mexico border, "mover(se)" and "mudar(se)" have the same meaning.

5. In the Spanish language, "ointment" is often literally translated to "ungüento." However, "ungüento" is an application that is based in water. An application based in oil is "pomada." However, people may interchange these words.

6. There are many different terms for "eyeglasses." The word "lentes" may be more common in northern Mexico, "anteojos" in southern Mexico, and "gafas" in South America.

7. The words "ophthalmalogist" and "optometrist" may be confusing when translated into Spanish. "Oculista" and "oftalmólogo" are persons or doctors who prescribe lenses. An "optometrista" is a technician who prepares the lenses.

Apuntes de gramática / Grammar notes

Reflexive verbs	Example: aplicar(se)	Aplíque**se** la pomada. Apply the ointment to yourself.
Indirect object (le)	Example: aplicar	Aplíque**le** la pomada a su hijo. Apply the ointment to your son.
Direct object (lo or la)		Aplíque**la** cuatro veces al día. Apply it (the ointment) four times a day.
Indirect object (se) + direct object (lo or la)		Aplíque**sela**. Apply it (the ointment) to him or her.

Ejercicios / Exercises

I. Haga las preguntas correspondientes a las siguientes respuestas. (Write questions that correspond to the following answers.)

1. _____

    Tengo muchas lagañas en los ojos, y por la mañana, despierto con los ojos pegados.

2. _____

    No me duelen pero me lloran mucho y los tengo muy irritados.

3. _____

    No, no he usado ninguna medicina, sólo me he lavado los ojos con manzanilla.

4. _____

    No, en general veo bien, pero me siguen supurando todo el día.

5. _____

    Sí, me dan unas punzadas muy fuertes en los oídos y también me supuran.

II. Complete las siguientes oraciones con las palabras adecuadas. (Complete the following sentences with the appropriate words.)

1. La _____ es una infección de los ojos que los hace _____.

2. La _____ es uno de los dolores más intensos que hay.

3. El glaucoma puede causar _____.

4. Un oído normal produce una cantidad adecuada de _____.

5. Las _____ salen en la orilla de los párpados y son muy dolorosas.

6. Si las personas tienen el oído enfermo pueden tener también _____ y _____.

III. Relacione las palabras con sus antónimos. (Relate the words with their antonyms.)

1._____ abrir   a. derecha

2._____ apretar   b. afuera

3._____ tibiar   c. muy poco

4._____ abajo   d. cerrar

5._____ izquierda   e. enfriar

6._____ antes   f. quitar

7._____ borroso   g. arriba

8._____ adentro   h. soltar

9._____ poner   i. claro

10._____ demasiado   j. después

IV. Complete las oraciones con la forma verbal apropiada. (Complete the sentences with the appropriate verb form.)

1. (haber, tener) ¿_____ _____ vértigo últimamente?

2. (deber, estar) El niño _____ _____ quieto por un rato después de que le ponga las gotas.

3. (tener que, oprimir) _____ _____ la lengüeta de la oreja después de aplicar las gotas.

4. No (haber, refrigerar) _____ _____ las gotas, por eso no las siente.

5. (deber, mantener) _____ _____ la punta del gotero o del tubo de pomada cerca del ojo, pero sin tocarlo.

V. Complete las oraciones con el mandato/subjuntivo. (Complete the sentences with the command/subjunctive form.)

1. (lavarse) El doctor quiere que usted _____ bien las manos.

2. (parpadear) Después de ponerse las gotas, _____ varias veces.

3. (mantener) Las instrucciones dicen que _____ las gotas fuera del alcance de los niños.

4. (oprimirse) Quiero que usted _____ el lagrimal con un dedo.

5. (aplicarse) Usted _____ una gota tres veces al día.

VI. Practique los verbos reflexivos y con el objeto directo e indirecto. (Practice using the verbs in reflexive form and with direct and indirect objects.)

1. (poner) Put the drops in your eye. _____

 Put the drops in his eye. _____

 Put them (the drops) in four times a day. _____

 Put the drops in her eyes. Put them in her. _____

2. (abrir) Open your eye with your fingers. _____

 Open his eye with your fingers. _____

 Open them (the eyes). _____

 Open the bottle for me. Open it for me. _____

REFERENCES

1. Fiscella RG, Jensen, MK. Ophthalmic disorders. In: Berardi RR, Kroon LA, McDermott JH, et al., eds. *Handbook of Nonprescription Drugs.* 15th ed. Washington, DC: American Pharmacists Association; 2006:577–603.

2. Gardner M, Boyce RW, Herrier RN. *Pharmacist–Patient Consultation Program PPCP-Unit I: An Interactive Approach to Verifying Patient Understanding.* New York: Pfizer Educational Services; 1991.

3. Lacy CF, Armstrong LL, Goldman MP, et al, eds. *Drug Information Handbook.* 17th ed. Hudson, Ohio: Lexi-comp, Inc; 2008.

4. Krypel L. Otic disorders. In: Berardi RR, Kroon LA, McDermott JH, et al., eds. *Handbook of Nonprescription Drugs.* 15th ed. Washington, DC: American Pharmacists Association; 2006:633–47.

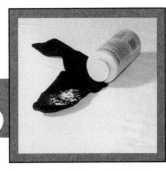

Productos para la piel
Skin products

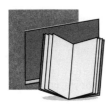

Lección 1 Pie de atleta
Lesson 1 Athlete's foot

Verbos / Verbs		Presente / Present tense			
		Yo	Él, ella, usted	Mandato	Ejemplos
cambiar(se)	to change	(me) cambio	(se) cambia	Cambie(se)	*Cámbiese los calcetines todas los días.*
curar(se)	to cure	(me) curo	(se) cura	Cure(se)	*Cúrese los pies con esta pomada.*
despellejar	to peel (skin)	se me despelleja	se le despelleja	—	*¿Se le despellejan los pies?*
oler	to smell	huelo	huele	Huela	*Los pies me huelen mal.*
producir	to produce	produzco	produce	Produzca	*La hiedra le produce ronchas.*
sangrar	to bleed	sangro	sangra	No sangre	*Algunas heridas sangran.*
secar(se)	to dry	(me) seco	(se) seca	Seque(se)	*Séquese bien los pies.*
tardar	to take time	tardo	tarda	Tarde	*La herida tarda dos días en curarse.*

Las partes del pie / Parts of the foot

el arco del pie	arch of the foot
los dedos de los pies	toes
el empeine del pie	top of the foot
la planta del pie	sole
el tobillo	ankle
las uñas de los pies	toe nails

Sustantivos / Nouns

el algodón	cotton
las calcetas	knee-highs
los calcetines	socks
el caso	case (situation)
el desecho	discharge
el engrosamiento	overgrowth
las escamas	scales (skin)
la(s) grieta(s)	cracking
el hongo	fungus
el olor	smell
la picazón	prickling
la pus	pus
la resequedad	dryness
las sandalias	sandals
la sensación	sensation
el talco	talc, powder
los zapatos	shoes

Adjetivos / Adjectives

adolorido(a)	sore
común	common
húmedo(a)	wet
seco(a)	dry
simple	simple
tópico(a)	topical

Otras expresiones / Other expressions

entre	between
muy común	very common
para uso externo	for external use
puede ser que	it might be that

Otros problemas de los pies / Other foot problems

las ampollas	blisters
el callo	corn, callus
el juanete	bunion
el mezquino	wart
el pie de atleta	athlete's foot
la uña enterrada	ingrown toenail

Otros problemas de la piel / Other skin problems*

la caspa	dandruff
la dermatitis	dermatitis
el(los) grano(s)	bump(s) (little growths)
la hiedra venenosa	poison ivy (plant)
la intoxicación con hiedra	poison ivy (problem)
el lunar	mole
la(s) peca(s)	freckle(s)
la piel reseca	dry skin
la rozadura de pañal	diaper rash
el salpullido, el sarpullido	rash
la supuración	oozing
la urticaria	urticaria

Las lesiones / Lesions*

la cortadura, la cortada	cut
la herida	wound
la lesión	lesion
el moretón	bruise
la quemadura	burn
la quemadura de sol	sunburn
la raspadura, el raspón	scratch

Las picaduras de insecto / Insect bites*

la picadura de abeja	bee sting
el piquete de mosquito	mosquito bite
la reacción	reaction
las ronchas	hives

Presentaciones / Formulations

el aceite	oil
el aerosol	spray
la avena	oatmeal
el bloqueador de sol	sunblock
el bronceador	suntan lotion
el champú	shampoo
la crema	cream, lotion
el curita	bandage
el gel	gel
el jabón	soap
la loción	lotion (facial), cologne
la loción limpiadora	cleanser
la pomada	ointment, cream
el protector solar	sunscreen
el talco	powder
el ungüento	ointment, cream
la vaselina	petroleum jelly, Vaseline®

Infecciones de la piel / Skin infections*

el herpes zoster	shingles
el impétigo	impetigo
la roña	scabies (common)
la rubéola	rubella
el sarampión	measles
la sarna	scabies (technical)
la varicela	chicken pox

*These vocabulary words are related to skin problems and are listed for reference.

Preguntas[1]

1. ¿Dónde, exactamente, tiene el problema? ¿Entre los dedos? ¿En la planta del pie?
2. ¿Tiene comezón en los pies? ¿Le huelen mal los pies?
3. ¿Tiene engrosamiento de la piel en los pies? ¿Tiene inflamación o enrojecimiento?
4. ¿Tiene escamas en los pies o se le despellejan? ¿Tiene pus o algún otro desecho? ¿De qué color?
5. ¿Le sangran los pies? ¿Le arden? ¿Tiene grietas?

Recomendaciones

El pie de atleta lo produce un hongo. Es una infección muy común.

Usted tiene un caso de pie de atleta ligero. Le recomiendo que use un talco medicinal.

Este talco contiene tolnaftate al 1%.

1. Mantenga sus pies limpios y secos. Lávese y séquese los pies.
2. Aplíquese el talco en los pies y en los zapatos dos veces al día.
3. Puede ser que después necesite una pomada tópica.
4. Puede tardar de 2 a 4 semanas en curarse el pie de atleta.

Recomendaciones adicionales

1. Cámbiese los calcetines todos los días. Use calcetines de algodón.
2. Evite tener los pies húmedos.
3. Es para uso externo solamente.

Efectos secundarios (molestias)

Puede sentir una picazón muy ligera en los pies o una sensación de ardor.

Las preguntas fundamentales[2]

1. ¿Para qué es esta medicina?
2. ¿Cómo va a aplicarse esta medicina?
3. ¿Cuáles son los efectos secundarios?
4. Quiero estar seguro(a) de que no olvidé nada. Por favor, dígame cómo va a usar esta medicina.

Questions[1]

1. Where exactly is the fungus on your feet? Between your toes? On the soles of your feet?
2. Do your feet itch? Do they smell bad?
3. Do you have a skin overgrowth on your feet? Is there inflammation or reddening?
4. Do you have scales on your feet or are they peeling? Is there pus or another discharge? What color?
5. Do your feet bleed? Do they burn? Do you have cracking?

Recommendations

Athlete's foot is a fungus. It is a very common infection.
You have a mild case of athlete's foot. I recommend a medicinal powder.
This powder contains tolnaftate 1%.

1. Keep your feet clean and dry. Wash and dry your feet.
2. Apply this powder to your feet and shoes twice a day.
3. You may need a topical cream (ointment) later.
4. It may take 2 to 4 weeks to cure the athlete's foot.

Additional recommendations

1. Change your socks every day. Wear cotton socks.
2. Avoid having your feet wet.
3. It's for external use only.

Side effects

Your feet may feel a light stinging or burning sensation.

Prime questions[2]

1. What is this medication for?
2. How are you going to apply this medication?
3. What are the side effects?
4. I want to be sure that I didn't forget anything. Please tell me how you are going to use this medicine.

Diálogos para el audio

FARMACÉUTICO: Buenos días. Soy el Dr. John Baker. ¿En qué le puedo servir?

PACIENTE: *Buenos días, doctor. Soy Lalo Quiñones. Pues, últimamente he tenido mucha comezón en los pies.*

FARMACÉUTICO: ¿Practica algún deporte?

PACIENTE: *Acabo de formar con mis amigos un equipo de fútbol.*

FARMACÉUTICO: ¡Que bueno! Quisiera hacerle algunas preguntas.

Preguntas[1]

1. ¿Dónde, exactamente, tiene el problema? ¿Entre los dedos? ¿En la planta del pie?
Entre los dedos y en la planta del pie también.

2. ¿Tiene comezón en los pies? ¿Le huelen mal los pies?
Tengo mucha comezón y también me huelen muy mal los pies y los zapatos.

3. ¿Tiene engrosamiento de la piel en los pies? ¿Tiene inflamación o enrojecimiento?
No tengo engrosamiento, pero si tengo los pies muy enrojecidos.

4. ¿Tiene escamas en los pies o se le despellejan? ¿Tiene pus o algún otro desecho? ¿De qué color?
Se me despellejan los pies, pero no tengo pus ni ningún otro deshecho.

5. ¿Le sangran los pies? ¿Le arden? ¿Tiene grietas?
Tengo algunas grietas entre los dedos y me arden mucho, pero no me sangran.

Recomendaciones

Creo que usted tiene un caso ligero de pie de atleta. El pie de atleta lo produce un hongo. Es una infección muy común. Le recomiendo que use un talco medicinal. Este talco contiene tolnaftate al 1%.

Para usar esta medicina:

1. Mantenga sus pies limpios y secos. Lávese y séquese los pies antes de aplicarse la medicina.

2. Aplíquese el talco en los pies y en los zapatos dos veces al día.

3. Puede ser que después necesite una pomada tópica.

4. Puede tardar de 2 a 4 semanas en curarse el pie de atleta.

Recomendaciones adicionales

1. También, use calcetines de algodón y cámbieselos todos los días.

2. Evite tener los pies húmedos.

3. Es para uso externo solamente.

Efectos secundarios (molestias)

Este talco puede causarle una picazón muy ligera en los pies o una sensación de ardor.

Las preguntas fundamentales[2]

1. Quiero estar seguro de que no olvidé nada. Dígame ¿Para qué es esta medicina?
Es para el pie de atleta que tengo.

2. ¿Cómo va a aplicarse esta medicina?
Me la voy a poner dos veces al día, después de lavarme y secarme muy bien los pies.

3. ¿Cuáles son los efectos secundarios?
Puede causarme una ligera picazón o ardor.

Muy bien. Pues, que se alivie pronto.

Gracias, doctor. Hasta luego.

Audio dialogues

PHARMACIST: Good morning. I am Dr. John Baker. How can I help you?

PATIENT: *Good morning, Doctor. I am Lalo Quiñones. Well, recently I have had a lot of itchiness in my feet.*

PHARMACIST: Do you practice (play) a sport?

PATIENT: *I just formed a soccer team with my friends.*

PHARMACIST: Oh, good! I would like to ask you a few questions.

Questions[1]

1. Where exactly is the problem? Between your toes? On the soles of your feet?
   Between my toes and on my soles, also.

2. Do your feet itch? Do they smell bad?
   I have a lot of itchiness in my feet, and also my feet and shoes smell very bad.

3. Do you have a skin overgrowth on your feet? Is there inflammation or reddening?
   No, I don't have overgrowth, but my feet are very red.

4. Do you have scales on your feet or are they peeling? Do you have pus or another discharge? What color?
   Yes, my feet are peeling, but I don't have pus or any other discharge.

5. Do your feet bleed? Do they burn? Do you have cracking?
   I have some cracking between the toes, and they burn a lot, but they don't bleed.

Recommendations

I believe that you have a mild case of athlete's foot. Athlete's foot produces a fungus. It is a very common infection. I recommend (to you) that you use a medicinal powder. This powder contains tolnaftate 1%.

To use this medicine
1. Keep your feet clean and dry. Wash and dry your feet before applying the medicine (to yourself).

2. Apply (to yourself) the powder to your feet and shoes two times a day.
3. It may be that you will need a topical cream later.
4. It may take 2 to 4 weeks to cure (yourself) of the athlete's foot.

Additional recommendations

1. Also, wear cotton socks and change them every day.
2. Avoid having your feet wet.
3. It is for external use only.

Side effects

This powder may cause you a light stinging or burning sensation in your feet.

Prime questions[2]

1. I want to be sure that I didn't forget anything. Tell me, what is this medication for?
   It is for the athlete's foot that I have.

2. How are you going to apply this medication (to yourself)?
   I am going to apply it (to myself) twice a day after washing and drying my feet very well.

3. What are the side effects?
   It can cause (me) a light stinging or burning.

Very good. Well, may you feel better soon.

Thank you, Doctor. Until later.

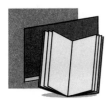

Lección 2   Acné
Lesson 2   Acne

Verbos / Verbs   Presente / Present tense

	Yo	Él, ella, usted	Mandato	Ejemplos
proteger — to protect	protejo	protege	Proteja	*Proteja su cara del sol.*
quemar(se) — to burn	(me) quemo	(se) quema	No (se) queme	*Puede quemarse si no usa bloqueador.*
rasurar(se) — to shave	(me) rasuro	(se) rasura	Rasure(se)	*Rasúrese con esta crema.*
resecar — to dry out	—	reseca	—	*La loción me reseca mucho.*

Las partes de cuerpo relacionadas con el acné / Body parts related to acne

la boca	mouth
el cuello	neck
la espalda	back
los labios	lips
el pecho	chest
la piel	skin

Sustantivos / Nouns

el acné	acne
el barro	blackhead
la capa	layer
la(s) espinilla(s)	pimple(s)
la loción para después de rasurarse (afeitarse)	after-shave lotion
el maquillaje	makeup
el punto blanco	whitehead
el punto negro	blackhead
la resequedad	dryness
el tipo	type

Adjetivos / Adjectives

afectado(a)	affected
alérgico(a)	allergic
delgado(a)	thin
grasoso(a)	oily
ligero(a)	light
reseco(a)	very dry
seco(a)	dry

Preguntas[3]
1. ¿Desde cuándo tiene acné?
2. ¿Qué tan seguido se lava la cara?
3. ¿Qué tipo de maquillaje usa usted?
4. ¿Qué tipo de loción para después de rasurarse (afeitarse) usa usted?
5. ¿Está usando algún tipo de medicamento para el acné?

Instrucciones
Benzoyl peroxide 2.5% (Peróxido benzoico al dos punto cinco por ciento)
1. Lávese la cara (o la piel) con agua y jabón neutro.
2. Aplíquese una capa muy delgada de esta crema en la parte afectada de una a tres veces al día.
3. Aplíquese el medicamento antes de ponerse el maquillaje.
4. Puede usarlo para prevenir nuevos barros y espinillas.
5. Evite aplicárselo en los párpados y los labios.

Efectos secundarios (molestias)
Puede causarle resequedad en la piel.

Recomendaciones adicionales
1. Proteja su cara del sol. Durante el día, use un protector solar.
2. Para uso externo solamente.

Las preguntas fundamentales[2]
1. ¿Para qué es esta medicina?
2. ¿Cómo va a aplicar esta medicina?
3. ¿Cuáles son los efectos secundarios?
4. Quiero estar seguro(a) de que no olvidé nada. Por favor, dígame cómo va a usar esta medicina.

Questions[3]

1. How long have you had acne?
2. How often do you wash your face?
3. What type of makeup do you use?
4. What type of aftershave do you use?
5. Are you using any acne medication now?

Directions

Benzoyl peroxide 2.5%

1. Wash your face (or your [affected] skin) with water and a neutral soap.
2. Apply (to yourself) a thin layer of this cream to the affected area one to three times a day.
3. Apply this medication (to yourself) before putting on makeup.
4. You may use it to prevent new blackheads and pimples.
5. Avoid applying it to the eyelids and lips.

Side effects

It may cause (you) dry skin.

Additional recommendations

1. Protect your face from the sun. During the day, use sunscreen.
2. For external use only.

Prime questions[2]

1. What is this medication for?
2. How are you going to apply this medication?
3. What are the side effects?
4. I want to be sure that I didn't forget anything. Please tell me how you are going to use this medicine.

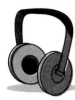

Diálogos para el audio

FARMACÉUTICA: Buenos días, me llamo Miriam Bates. ¿Cómo le puedo ayudar?

PACIENTE: *Buenos días, Srta. Bates. Soy Angélica Gómez. Pues, tengo muchos barros y espinillas y tengo la cara muy grasosa. Y ahora, cuando me rasuro las piernas, me salen granitos. ¿Me puede recomendar algo para estos problemas? Tengo que ir a una fiesta el viernes, y no quiero tener así la cara ni las piernas porque se ve muy feo.*

FARMACÉUTICA: Sí, desde luego. Pero primero quiero hacerle algunas preguntas. ¿Cuántos años tiene?

PACIENTE: *Acabo de cumplir 14 años.*

Preguntas[3]

1. ¿Desde cuándo tiene acné?
   Pues, más o menos desde hace un mes.

2. ¿Qué tan seguido se lava la cara?
   Me la lavo dos veces al día, en la mañana y en la noche.

3. ¿Qué tipo de maquillaje usa?
   Uso un maquillaje en crema.

4. ¿Usa algún tipo de loción después de rasurarse las piernas?
   Nada más uso jabón para rasurarme. No uso cremas ni lociones.

5. ¿Está usando algún tipo de medicamento para el acné?
   Pues, he usado algunas cremas, pero no me han dado resultado.

Bueno pues, le voy a recomendar un medicamento muy bueno para el acné.

Instrucciones

Esta crema contiene peróxido benzoico 2.5% (al dos punto cinco por ciento). Le va a resecar un poco la piel de la cara, pero no se preocupe. Le va a curar el acné.

1. Antes de usarla, lávese la cara con agua y un jabón neutro que no tenga perfume.
2. Aplíquese una capa muy delgada de esta crema en los barros y las espinillas de una a tres veces al día.
3. Aplíquese la crema antes de ponerse el maquillaje. Use un maquillaje líquido, no en crema.
4. También, puede usarla para prevenir nuevos barros y espinillas.
5. No se la aplique en los párpados ni en los labios.

Efectos secundarios (molestias)

La crema puede causarle un poco de resequedad en la piel.

Recomendaciones adicionales

1. Proteja su cara del sol. Cuando salga afuera, use un protector solar. Siempre use un sombrero o una gorra.
2. Esta crema es para uso externo solamente.
3. Para las piernas, use una crema sin perfume después de rasurarse para evitar los granitos.

Las preguntas fundamentales[2]

Para confirmar que le expliqué bien, dígame . . .

1. ¿Para qué es esta crema?
   Es para tratar el acné.

2. ¿Cómo va a aplicarse esta crema?
   Me voy a aplicar una capa muy delgada en los barros y las espinillas todo el día entre las clases.

   ¡No, por favor! ¡Solamente de una a tres veces al día o le puede resecar demasiado la cara!

3. ¿Cuáles son las molestias que le puede causar la crema?
   Pues, me puede causar resequedad en la cara.

4. Quiero estar segura de que no olvidé nada. Por favor, dígame cómo va a usar esta medicina.
   Me la voy a aplicar de una a tres veces al día.

Sí, muy bien. Pues, espero que se cure rápido con la crema y que disfrute mucho de la fiesta.

Ay, muchas gracias, señorita. Usted me ayudó mucho porque quiero verme muy bien.

Audio dialogues

PHARMACIST: Good morning, my name is Miriam Bates. How can I help you?

PATIENT: *Good morning, Miss Bates. I am Angélica Gómez. Well, I have a lot of blackheads and pimples, and I have a very oily face. And now, when I shave my legs, I get little bumps (erupt). Can you recommend (to me) something for these problems? I have to go to a party on Friday, and I don't want to have my face or my legs like this because it looks really ugly.*

PHARMACIST: Yes, of course. But first I want to ask you a few questions. How old are you?

PATIENT: *I just turned 14 years old.*

Questions[3]

1. How long have you had acne?
   Well, more or less about a month.

2. How often do you wash your face?
   I wash it twice a day, in the morning and at night.

3. What type of makeup do you use?
   I use a cream makeup.

4. Do you use some type of lotion after shaving your legs?
   I only use soap to shave (myself). I don't use any creams or lotions.

5. Are you using any acne medication now?
   Well, I have used some creams, but they have not worked.

Well then, I am going to recommend (to you) a very good medication for your acne.

Directions

This cream contains benzoyl peroxide 2.5%. It will dry out your face a little bit, but don't worry. It will help (cure) your acne.

1. Before using it, wash your face with water and a neutral soap that doesn't have perfume.
2. Apply (to yourself) a thin layer of this cream on the blackheads and pimples one to three times a day.
3. Apply (to yourself) the cream before putting on makeup. Use a liquid makeup, not cream.
4. Also, you may use it to prevent new blackheads and pimples.
5. Don't apply it to your eyelids or lips.

Side effects

The cream may cause (you) a little dry skin.

Additional recommendations

1. Protect your face from the sun. When you go outside, use sunscreen. Always use a hat or baseball cap.
2. This cream is for external use only.
3. For your legs, use a cream without perfume after shaving (yourself) to avoid little bumps.

Prime questions[2]

To confirm that I explained it well (to you), tell me . . .
1. What is this cream for?
   It is for the acne.

2. How are you going to apply this cream (to yourself)?
   I am going to apply a very thin layer on my blackheads and pimples all day between classes.

   No, please! Only one to three times a day, or it can dry your face out too much!

3. What are the side effects the cream can cause you?
   Well, it can cause (me) dry skin on the face.

4. I want to be sure that I didn't forget anything. Please, tell me how you are going to use this medicine.
   I am going to apply it one to three times a day.

Yes, very good. Well, I hope you get better fast with the cream and that you enjoy the party.

Oh, many thanks, miss. You helped me so much because I want to look very nice.

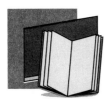

Lección 3 Los piojos
Lesson 3 Lice

Verbos / Verbs		Presente / Present tense			
		Yo	Él, ella, usted	Mandato	Ejemplos
aspirar	to vacuum	aspiro	aspira	Aspire	*Aspire las alfombras.*
contagiar(se)	to get infected	(me) contagio	(se) contagia	No (se) contagie	*El niño se contagió en la escuela.*
dejar	to leave	dejo	deja	Deje	*Déjele el champú 10 minutos.*
desinfectar	to disinfect	desinfecto	desinfecta	Desinfecte	*Desinfecte la ropa.*
enjuagar(se)	to rinse	(me) enjuago	(se) enjuaga	Enjuague(se)	*Enjuáguese el cabello después de lavarlo.*
matar	to kill	mato	mata	Mate	*Mate los piojos y liendres con este medicamento.*
peinar(se)	to comb	(me) peino	(se) peina	Peine(se)	*Péinese con un peine de dientes finos.*
rascar(se)	to scratch	(me) rasco	(se) rasca	Rasque(se)	*No se rasque las ronchas.*
remojar	to soak	remojo	remoja	Remoje	*Remoje los cepillos en agua muy caliente.*
tirar	to dispose of (to throw away)	tiro	tira	Tire	*Tírelas a la basura.*
usar	to use	uso	usa	Use	*No use peines de otras personas.*

Las partes de la cabeza / Parts of the head

el cabello	hair
el cuero cabelludo	scalp
el pelo	hair

Sustantivos / Nouns

el abrigo	coat
la bufanda	scarf
la cachucha	cap (baseball)
el casco	helmet
el cepillo	brush

el ciclo	cycle
el crisantemo	chrysanthemum
la gorra	cap (baseball)
el peine	comb
el sombrero	hat

Adjetivos / Adjectives

cerrado(a)	closed
húmedo(a)	damp
infectado(a)	infected
muerto(a)	dead

Otras expresiones / Other expressions

bien caliente	very hot
de dientes muy finos	fine-toothed
la ropa de cama	bed linens

Preguntas[4]

1. ¿Hay otras personas en la familia que tengan piojos?
2. ¿Ultimamente, hay alguien se rasca mucho la cabeza (en la familia, entre los amigos)?

Instrucciones

Los piojos son muy comunes. Probablemente su hijo(a) se contagió en la escuela. Le recomiendo que use un champú medicinal. Es un champú que contiene permethrin al 1% (uno por ciento).

1. Aplíquele el champú en la cabeza hasta que todo el pelo esté húmedo.
2. Déjele el champú durante 10 (diez) minutos.
3. Haga una espuma con agua tibia.
4. Lávele el cabello después con champú normal.
5. Enjuágueselo muy bien.
6. Use un peine de dientes muy finos para quitar los piojos muertos y las liendres.
7. Repita el tratamiento en 7 a 10 días para matar cualquier piojo nuevo.

Recomendaciones adicionales

1. Si el (la) paciente es alérgico a los crisantemos o al "ragweed," necesitará otro tipo de productos.
2. Es para uso externo solamente.
3. Aplíqueles el mismo tratamiento a todas las personas que vivan en la casa.

Recomendaciones para desinfectar la casa

1. Lave la ropa de cama y la ropa de la persona infectada en la lavadora con agua bien caliente.
2. Desinfecte bien las cosas de la cabeza (por ejemplo, los sombreros, las gorras, los cascos, las bufandas y los abrigos).
3. Use el ciclo más caliente de la secadora (cuando seque la ropa y la ropa de cama).
4. Remoje los peines y los cepillos en agua bien caliente y lávelos.
5. Aspire los cuartos muy bien. Tire la bolsa de la aspiradora inmediatamente.
6. Ponga las otras cosas que no se puedan lavar (por ejemplo, los cojines, las almohadas o los muñecos de peluche) en una bolsa de plástico cerrada, por lo menos durante 2 semanas.
7. Si puede, tire todas las cosas que estén infectadas.

Las preguntas fundamentales[2]

1. ¿Para qué es esta medicina?
2. ¿Cómo va a aplicar este champú?
3. Quiero estar seguro(a) que no olvidé nada. Por favor, dígame cómo va a usar esta medicina.

Questions[4]

1. Are there other people in the family who have lice?
2. Lately, is there anyone who scratches his (her) head a lot (in the family, among friends)?

Directions

Lice are very common. Your son (daughter) probably contracted the lice at school. I recommend you use this medicated shampoo. This shampoo contains permethrin 1%.

1. Apply the shampoo to his (her) head until all the hair is damp.
2. Leave the shampoo on his (her) hair for 10 minutes.
3. Lather with warm water.
4. Wash his (her) hair with a normal shampoo afterward.
5. Rinse it (his or her hair) very well.
6. Use a fine-toothed comb to remove dead lice and the eggs (nits).
7. Repeat the treatment in 7 to 10 days to kill any newly hatched lice.

Additional recommendations

1. If the patient is allergic to chrysanthemums or ragweed, he (she) will need another type of product.
2. (It is) for external use only.
3. Apply (to themselves) the same treatment to all of the people who live in the house.

Recommendations to disinfect the house

1. Wash bed linens and the clothing of the infected person in a washing machine with very hot water.
2. Disinfect items for the head (for example, hats, baseball caps, helmets, scarves, and coats).
3. Use the hottest dryer cycle (when drying clothes and sheets).
4. Soak combs and brushes in very hot water and wash them.
5. Vacuum rooms very well. Throw away the vacuum bag immediately.
6. Put other things that you cannot wash (for example, cushions, pillows, or stuffed animals) in a closed plastic bag for at least 2 weeks.
7. If you can, throw away all the things that might be infected.

Prime questions[2]

1. What is this medication for?
2. How are you going to apply this shampoo?
3. I want to be sure that I didn't forget anything. Please tell me how you are going to use this medicine.

Diálogos para el audio

FARMACÉUTICO: Buenos días, me llamo Ed Barker. ¿En qué le puedo servir?

PACIENTE: *Buenos días, Sr. Barker. Soy la Sra. Pérez. Sabe que mi hija se contagió de piojos en la escuela y necesito alguna medicina segura para tratar el problema.*

FARMACÉUTICO: Por supuesto, pero primero quisiera hacerle algunas preguntas.

Preguntas[4]

¿Hay otras personas en la familia que tengan piojos?
¿Hay alguien que se rasque mucho la cabeza?
Creo que sí porque he visto que mi hijo se rasca mucho la cabeza. Sin embargo, no lo he revisado. Tal vez tenga que darles el tratamiento a los dos.

Sí, le recomiendo que revise bien al niño, y si tiene piojos también póngale la medicina. Esta medicina no es tomada—no se la dé a sus hijos por la boca. Esta medicina es un champú. Solamente es para uso externo. Pídale a otra persona que les revise la cabeza a todas las personas que viven en la casa porque los piojos son muy contagiosos.
Ah. Gracias por clarificarme. ¿Qué más me aconseja?

Instrucciones

Pues, los piojos son muy comunes. Probablemente su hija se contagió en la escuela. Le voy a recomendar un champú medicinal. Es un champú que contiene permethrin al 1%.

1. Aplíquele a su hija el champú en la cabeza hasta que todo el pelo esté húmedo. Haga lo mismo con sus otros hijos si también ellos tienen piojos. Los adultos deben seguir las mismas instrucciones.
2. Déjele el medicamento durante 10 minutos.
3. Haga una espuma con agua tibia.
4. Lávele el cabello después con champú normal.
5. Enjuágueselo muy bien.
6. Use un peine de dientes muy finos para quitar los piojos muertos y las liendres.
7. Repita el tratamiento en 7 a 10 días para matar cualquier piojo nuevo.

Recomendaciones adicionales

1. Si su hija es alérgica a los crisantemos o al "ragweed," necesitará otro tipo de productos.
2. Recuerde que es para uso externo solamente.

Recomendaciones para desinfectar la casa

También, le voy a hacer algunas recomendaciones para desinfectar toda la casa porque los piojos pueden infectar muchas cosas—son muy contagiosos.

1. Lave la ropa de cama y la ropa de las personas infectadas en la lavadora con agua bien caliente.
2. Desinfecte las cosas que hayan tenido contacto con la cabeza, por ejemplo, los sombreros, las gorras, los cascos, las bufandas y los abrigos.
3. Use el ciclo más caliente de la secadora cuando seque la ropa y la ropa de cama.
4. Remoje los peines y los cepillos en agua bien caliente y lávelos muy bien.
5. Aspire los cuartos muy bien. Tire la bolsa de la aspiradora inmediatamente.
6. Ponga las otras cosas que no se puedan lavar en una bolsa de plástico cerrada, por lo menos durante 2 semanas—por ejemplo, los cojines, las almohadas o los muñecos de peluche.
7. Si puede, tire todas las cosas que estén infectadas.

Las preguntas fundamentales[2]

Creo que las instrucciones son un poco complicadas. Entonces, quisiera confirmar como va a usar el medicamento. ¿Me puede decir la siguiente?

1. ¿Para qué es este champú?
   Es para matar los piojos.

2. ¿Cómo va a usar este champú?
   Lo voy a aplicar como un champú y dejarlo por 10 minutos. Después voy a lavarles la cabeza con champú normal. Voy a peinarlos con cuidado con un peine de dientes finos para sacarles los piojos y las liendres. Tengo que repetir el tratamiento en 7 a 10 días para matar los piojos nuevos.

3. Ah, muy bien. Quiero estar seguro que no olvidé nada. Por favor, dígame cómo va a usar esta medicina.
   Se la voy a aplicar directamente en la cabeza y la dejaré allí durante 10 minutos. También, tengo que desinfectar toda la ropa de cama y toda la casa.

Muy bien. Le voy a dar las instrucciones por escrito porque son muy complicadas.

Ay, muchísimas gracias, Sr. Barker.

Que le vaya bien.

Audio dialogues

PHARMACIST: Good morning, my name is Ed Barker. How can I serve you?

PATIENT: *Good morning, Mr. Barker. I am Mrs. Pérez. You know that my daughter contracted lice at school, and I need some safe medicine to treat the problem.*

PHARMACIST: Of course, but first I would like to ask you some questions.

Questions[4]

Are there other people in the family who have lice? Is there anyone who scratches (his or her) head a lot?
I think so, because I have seen that my son scratches his head a lot. However, I have not checked him. Perhaps I have to give (orally) the treatment to both of them.

Yes, I recommend that you check the boy very well, and if he has lice, also apply the medicine to him. This medicine is not taken orally—don't give your children the medicine by mouth. This medicine is a shampoo. It is only for external use. Ask another person to check the heads of all the people in your house because lice are very contagious.
Oh. Thank you for clarifying for me. What else can you advise (me)?

Directions

Well, lice are very common. Probably your daughter contracted the lice at school. I am going to recommend (to you) a medicated shampoo. It is a shampoo that contains permethrin 1%.

1. Apply the shampoo to your daughter's head until all of her hair is wet. Do the same with your other children if they also have lice. Adults should follow the same directions.
2. Leave it in her hair for 10 minutes.
3. Lather with warm water.
4. Wash her hair afterward with regular shampoo.
5. Rinse it (her hair) very well.
6. Use a fine-toothed comb to remove dead lice and the nits.
7. Repeat the treatment in 7 to 10 days to kill any newly hatched lice.

Additional recommendations

1. If your daughter is allergic to chrysanthemums or ragweed, she will need another type of product.
2. Remember that it is for external use only.

Recommendations to disinfect the house

Also, I am going to make some other recommendations to disinfect all of the house, because lice can infect many things—(they) are very contagious.

1. Wash bed linens and the clothes of the persons infected in a washing machine with very hot water.
2. Disinfect items that have been in contact with the head—for example, hats, baseball caps, helmets, scarves, and coats.
3. Use the hottest dryer cycle when drying clothes and sheets.
4. Soak combs and brushes in very hot water and wash them well.
5. Vacuum rooms very well. Throw away the vacuum bag immediately.
6. Put other things that you cannot wash in a closed plastic bag for at least 2 weeks—for example, cushions, pillows, or stuffed animals.
7. If you can, throw away the things that may be infected.

Prime questions[2]

I believe that the directions are a bit complicated. So I would like to confirm how you are going to use the medication. Can you tell me the following?

1. What is this shampoo for?
   It is to kill the lice.

2. How are you going to use this shampoo?
   I am going to apply it like a shampoo and leave it for 10 minutes. Later, I am going to wash their heads with a regular shampoo. I am going to comb them (their heads) carefully with a fine toothed comb to take out the lice and nits. I have to repeat the treatment in 7 to 10 days to kill the new lice.

3. Oh, very good. I want to be sure that I didn't forget anything. Please, tell me how you are going to use this medicine.
   I am going to apply it (medicine) to them directly on the head, and I will leave it (the medicine) for 10 minutes. Also, I have to disinfect the bed linens and all of the house.

Very good. I am going to give you written directions because they are very complicated.

Oh, thank you very much, Mr. Barker.

May all go well for you.

De la cultura / About the culture

1. Various treatments for skin problems are used in Mexico:
   a. Many people use cornstarch to relieve itching or hives caused by insect bites.
   b. In the case of a newborn's rash, people used to bathe the baby in water with an infusion of rose hips (rosa de castilla).
   c. People may apply petroleum to the head to cure lice. They also wash the head with a very strong detergent to cure fungus such as *tinea capitis*. Others prefer to shave the boy's head or give little girls a very short haircut.
2. It is very important to use the term "aplicar" or "poner" when referring to topical medications. The term "dar" in Spanish specifically refers to an oral administration. If you tell a parent to give (dar) his or her child a medication, the parent will give it to the child by mouth.
3. As in the United States, in Mexico it is embarrassing to have lice. However, it is very common for children to contract lice in schools or playgrounds. Many people have had lice at least once in their lives.
4. The term for "corn" as found on the feet is "callo." The term is not "maíz," which is the Spanish word for corn that is food.
5. The word "talco" is a powder or talc that is applied to the body. The term "polvo" refers to medicinal powders taken by mouth, powders that are mixed with water (e.g., antibiotic suspensions), powder used for makeup, and dust.

Apuntes de gramática / Grammar notes

Negative commands

When using negative commands, the verb is conjugated like regular commands (mandatos).
The "no" always goes before the conjugated verb.

Example: No use talco.   Don't use talcum powder.

Ejercicios / Exercises

I. Use oraciones completas para contestar las siguientes preguntas. (Use complete sentences to answer the following questions.)

1. Doctor, tengo la piel muy reseca. ¿Qué puedo hacer para suavizarla?

   _____

2. Doctor, mi hijo tiene piojos. ¿Qué puedo hacer?

   _____

3. Este fin de semana me picaron los mosquitos y tengo muchas ronchas. Por favor recomiéndeme algo para la comezón y las ronchas.

   _____

4. Tengo una comezón muy fuerte entre los dedos de los pies y me huelen mal. ¿Hay algún tratamiento para curarlos?

   _____

5. Mi bebé está muy rozado y llora mucho. ¿Cómo puedo curarlo?

   _____

6. Tengo barros y espinillas en la cara y en la espalda. ¿Son caras las cremas para el tratamiento de este problema?

   _____

7. Ayer fui a la playa y me quemé con el sol. La espalda y la cara me arden mucho. ¿Puede darme algo para curar la quemadura?

   _____

8. ¿Qué puedo hacer para no quemarme con el sol otra vez?

   _____

9. Tengo muchos callos en los pies. ¿Hay algún tratamiento para quitarlos?

   _____

10. ¿Para qué es un protector solar?

    _____

11. Me hice una cortadura muy grande en la mano. ¿Me pongo sólo un curita?

    _____

12. Creo que toqué hiedra venenosa porque tengo ronchas y picazón en la mano. También me arde y me duele mucho. ¿Qué me recomienda?

    _____

II. Llene los espacios en blanco con la palabra correcta. (Fill in the blanks with the correct word.)

1. La _____ es una resequedad de la piel que se puede curar con _____.

2. La _____ causada por la hiedra venenosa puede producir _____ y mucha _____.

3. _____ del _____ es un problema de los bebés que produce mucha irritación y dolor.

4. Los _____ son deformidades de los huesos de los pies.

5. Si las personas tienen _____ de _____ es mejor que usen calcetines de algodón y mantengan sus pies limpios y secos.

III. Relacione las siguientes palabras con la definición correcta. (Match the following words with the correct definitions.)

1. ___ quemadura   a. herida o cualquier otro tipo de daño en el cuerpo

2. ___ barros y espinillas   b. poner

3. ___ callo   c. lesión producida por exceso de calor

4. ___ lesión   d. engrosamiento de la piel

5. ___ aplicar   e. acné

6. ___ intoxicación   f. envenenamiento por algo externo al cuerpo

7. ___ tardar   g. tomar tiempo

8. ___ contagiarse   h. contraer una enfermedad por contacto de diferentes tipos

◼ Gramática / Grammar

IV. Construya mandatos negativos con las siguientes palabras. (Construct negative commands with the following words.)

1. Lavarse / el cabello / jabón

2. Rascarse / las ronchas

3. Salir / el sol

4. Poner / calcetines / poliéster

V. Complete las oraciones con la conjugación correcta de los verbos. (Complete the sentences with the correct conjugation of the verb.)

1. (haber, tener) Yo _____ _____ acné por muchos meses.

2. (tener que, mantener) Para curar el pie de atleta _____ _____ los pies muy limpios y secos.

3. (sangrar, tener) Si le _____ los pies, probablemente _____ pie de atleta.

4. (rascar[se], contagiar[se]) Los niños _____ mucho la cabeza cuando _____ de piojos.

REFERENCES

1. Newton GD, Popovich NG. Fungal skin infections. In: Berardi RR, Kroon LA, McDermott JH, et al., eds. *Handbook of Nonprescription Drugs*. 15th ed. Washington, DC: American Pharmacists Association; 2006:889–905.
2. Gardner M, Boyce RW, Herrier RN. *Pharmacist–Patient Consultation Program PPCP-Unit I: An Interactive Approach to Verifying Patient Understanding*. New York: Pfizer Educational Services; 1991.
3. Foster KT, Coffey CW. Acne. In: Berardi RR, Kroon LA, McDermott JH, et al., eds. *Handbook of Nonprescription Drugs*. 15th ed. Washington, DC: American Pharmacists Association; 2006:803–16.
4. Buff W, Fuhrman C. Insect Bites and Stings and Pediculosis. In: Berardi RR, Kroon LA, McDermott JH, et al., eds. *Handbook of Nonprescription Drugs*. 15th ed. Washington, DC: American Pharmacists Association; 2006:781–801.

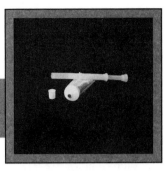

Capítulo 7 / Chapter 7

Productos vaginales y rectales
Vaginal and rectal products

Verbos / Verbs		Presente / Present tense			
		Yo	Él, ella, usted	Mandato	Ejemplos
acostar(se)	to lie (oneself) down, to go to bed	me acuesto	se acuesta	Acuéstese	*Acuéstese de lado.*
colocar	to place	coloco	coloca	Coloque	*Coloque la tapa al revés.*
conectar	to attach	conecto	conecta	Conecte	*Conecte el aplicador al tubo.*
depositar	to deposit	deposito	deposita	Deposite	*Deposite la crema dentro de la vagina.*
empujar	to push	empujo	empuja	Empuje	*Empuje el émbolo completamente.*
endurecer	to harden	endurezco	endurece	Endurezca	*El supositorio se endurece en el refrigerador.*
estar embarazada	to be pregnant	estoy embarazada	está embarazada	No se embarace	*No se embarace mientras use este medicamento.*
humedecer	to moisten, to wet	humedezco	humedece	Humedezca	*Humedezca el supositorio en agua tibia.*
introducir	to insert	introduzco	introduce	Introduzca	*Introduzca el óvulo suavemente.*
llenar	to fill with a volume	lleno	llena	Llene	*Llene el tubo con la crema.*
oprimir	to press, to squeeze	oprimo	oprime	Oprima	*Oprima el tubo de la crema.*
parar(se)	to stand (oneself)	me paro	se para	Párese	*Párese con las piernas separadas.*
retirar	to take away, to take out	retiro	retira	Retire	*Retire el aplicador.*
romper	to break, to tear	rompo	rompe	Rompa	*Rompa el sello protector.*

Los órganos genitales / Genital organs

Femenino	Female	Masculino	Male
el cervix	cervix	el escroto	scrotum
los genitales femeninos	female genitals	los genitales masculinos	male genitals
el ovario	ovary	el pene, el miembro	penis
la pelvis	pelvis	la próstata	prostate
las trompas de Falopio	fallopian tubes	el testículo	testicle
la uretra	urethra	la uretra	urethra
el útero o la matriz	uterus	las vesículas seminales	seminal vesicles
la vagina	vagina		
la vulva	vulva		

Sustantivos / Nouns

el agua tibia	lukewarm water
el antiséptico	antiseptic
el aplicador	applicator
el área	area
el desecho	discharge
el flujo vaginal	vaginal discharge
el embarazo	pregnancy
el émbolo	plunger (applicator part)
la envoltura	wrapper
la etiqueta	label
el hongo	fungus
el óvulo	vaginal suppository
las partes privadas (genitales)	private parts (genitals)
el producto	product
la regla (menstruación, período)	menstruation
el sello	seal
el supositorio	suppository
el tampón	tampon
la tapa	lid
la toalla sanitaria	sanitary pad
el tubo	tube

Adjetivos / Adjectives

blanco(a)	white
blando(a)	soft
blancuzco(a)	whitish
desechable	disposable
doblado(a)	bent, folded
espeso(a)	thick
tibio(a)	lukewarm

Otras expresiones / Other expressions

al revés	backward, opposite side
antes y después	before and after
boca arriba	on your back or face up
boca abajo	lying with your face down
el dedal de hule	finger cot (rubber)
de lado	on your side
(a)dentro	inside
ligeramente	slightly, lightly
el papel higiénico, el papel sanitario	toilet paper
sólo, solamente	only
suavemente	gently

La salud sexual / Sexual health

el aborto natural, el malparto	miscarriage
el aborto provocado	abortion (induced)
el cáncer de la matriz	uterine cancer
el cáncer del seno	breast cancer
el cáncer testicular	testicular cancer
la disfunción eréctil	erectile dysfunction
el(la) ginecólogo(a)	gynecologist
el herpes genital	genital herpes
el papanicolau	Pap smear
el prurito de los jockeys	jock itch
el SIDA (síndrome de inmuno-deficiencia adquirida)	AIDS (acquired immuno-deficiency syndrome)
el VIH (virus de immuno-deficiencia humana)	HIV (human immuno-deficiency virus)
el VPH (virus del papiloma humano)	HPV (human papilloma virus)

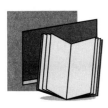

Lección 1   Productos vaginales
Lesson 1   Vaginal products

Preguntas[1]

1. ¿Cuáles son sus síntomas? ¿Qué síntomas tiene?
   — ¿Tiene comezón (en sus partes privadas: la vagina o la vulva o en ambas)?
   — ¿Hay algún desecho o flujo? ¿Es blanco o espeso?
   — ¿Hay enrojecimiento (vulvar o vaginal)?
   — ¿Tiene irritación (vulvar o vaginal)?
   — ¿Le duele (el área genital o sus partes privadas)?
   — ¿Tiene mal olor (en el área genital o en sus partes privadas)?
2. ¿Ha tenido algún tipo de infección vaginal en otras ocasiones?
3. ¿Desde cuándo tiene los síntomas?
4. ¿Está tomando medicamentos o está usando alguna crema para la vagina?
5. ¿Está usando algún antibiótico?

Recomendación

Miconazole en crema al 4% (cuatro por ciento)
Esta medicina es para la infección vaginal producida por un hongo. Es una crema que se aplica en la vagina. Aplíquese la crema dentro de la vagina por las noches durante tres días.

Efectos secundarios (molestias)

Esta medicina le puede causar ardor, comezón o irritación.

Instrucciones

1. Lávese bien las manos con agua y jabón antes y después de aplicarse la medicina.
2. Lávese y séquese el área genital.
3. Abra el tubo (así). (Más específico: Coloque la tapa al revés en el tubo para romper el sello.)
4. Conecte el aplicador al tubo.
5. Oprima (Apriete) el tubo para llenar el aplicador con la crema.
6. Acuéstese boca arriba con las piernas separadas y dobladas. O si quiere, párese con los pies separados y las rodillas ligeramente dobladas.
7. Suavemente introduzca todo el aplicador dentro de la vagina.
8. Empuje el émbolo para depositar la crema dentro de la vagina.
9. Retire el aplicador y después lávelo y enjuáguelo muy bien.
10. Si el aplicador es desechable tírelo a la basura.

Consejos adicionales

1. Puede usar una toalla sanitaria mientras esté usando la medicina. No use tampones.
2. Puede usar la medicina también durante los días de su regla.
3. Durante el embarazo, hable con su doctor.

Vía de administración

Sólo para uso vaginal

Las preguntas fundamentales[2]

1. ¿Para qué es esta medicina?
2. ¿Cómo va a aplicar esta medicina?
3. ¿Cuáles son los efectos secundarios?
4. Quiero confirmar que no se me olvidó nada. Por favor, dígame cómo va a usar esta medicina.

Questions[1]

1. What are your symptoms? What symptoms do you have?
   — Do you have itching (in your private parts: vagina, vulva, or both)?
   — Is there some discharge (or more fluid discharge)? Is it white or thick?
   — Is there redness (vulvar or vaginal)?
   — Do you have irritation (vulvar or vaginal)?
   — Does it (the genital area or private parts) hurt?
   — Do you have a bad odor (in the genital area or in your private parts)?
2. Have you had other types of vaginal infections in the past?
3. How long have you had the symptoms?
4. Are you taking medications or using a cream for the vaginal area?
5. Are you using an antibiotic?

Recommendation

Miconazole cream 4%

This medicine is for a vaginal infection caused by a fungus. It is a cream used vaginally. Insert cream into vagina at night for 3 days.

Side effects

This medicine may cause burning, itching, or irritation.

Directions

1. Wash your hands well with water and soap before and after inserting the medicine.
2. Wash and dry the genital area.
3. Open the tube (like this). (More specifically: Place the cap backward in the tube to break the seal.)
4. Attach the applicator to the tube.
5. Squeeze the tube to fill the applicator with cream.
6. Lie on your back with knees bent and open, or stand with your feet slightly apart and knees bent.
7. Gently insert the entire applicator into the vagina.
8. Push the plunger in to deposit cream into the vagina.
9. Remove the applicator and wash and rinse it very well.
10. If it is a disposable applicator, throw it away.

Other advice

1. You may use a sanitary pad while using the medicine. Do not use tampons.
2. You may also use the medicine during the days of your menstruation.
3. During pregnancy, talk to your doctor.

Administration route

For vaginal use only

Prime questions[2]

1. What is the medication for?
2. How are you going to apply the medication?
3. What are the side effects?
4. I want to make sure that I didn't forget anything. Please, tell me how you are going to use this medicine.

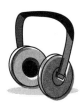

Diálogos para el audio

FARMACÉUTICA: Buenos días. Soy Janet Harris, la farmacéutica. ¿Cómo la puedo ayudar?

PACIENTE: *Mucho gusto, Dra. Harris. Buenos días. Soy Ana Ramos y necesito que me recomiende algún producto efectivo . . . pues traigo mucha irritación en mi . . . bueno, usted ya sabe, . . . allá abajo, es decir en mis partes privadas . . . en la vagina. Me da mucha pena y no sé qué ponerme. Tengo mucha comezón.*

FARMACÉUTICA: Lo siento, Srta. Ramos, pero no le dé pena. Este problema es muy común. Vamos a ver. Primero debo hacerle algunas preguntas antes de recomendarle un producto para tratar el problema.

PACIENTE: *Ah, claro. Entiendo.*

Preguntas[1]

1. ¿Cuáles son sus síntomas?
   Siento irritación, ardor, mucha picazón.
   ¿Tiene comezón en su área vaginal?
   Ay, sí.
   ¿Tiene flujo o hay algún desecho?
   Sí, tengo un poco de flujo.
   ¿Es blanco o espeso?
   Sí, es blancuzco.
   ¿Hay enrojecimiento?
   Creo que sí. También siento inflamación.
   ¿Tiene irritación?
   Sí, toda el área está irritada.
   ¿Le duele?
   Sí, algo. Me siento muy incómoda.
   ¿Ha notado mal olor en el flujo o en sus partes privadas?
   No, no creo.

2. ¿Ha tenido algún tipo de infección vaginal en otras ocasiones?
   Sí, hace 3 años.

3. ¿Desde cuándo tiene los síntomas?
   Desde antier.

4. ¿Está tomando medicamentos o está usando alguna crema para el área genital?
   No, no estoy usando nada.

5. ¿Está usando o tomando algún antibiótico?
   No, ninguna medicina.

6. ¿Está embarazada o piensa quedar embarazada en estos días?
   No, creo que no estoy embarazada y estoy tomando anticonceptivos para evitar el embarazo.

Recomendaciones

Ah, bueno. Le voy a recomendar miconazole en crema al 4% (cuatro por ciento). Esta medicina es para tratar la infección vaginal producida por un hongo. Es una crema que se aplica en la vagina. Aplíquese la crema dentro de la vagina durante 3 días antes de acostarse. Si no ve una mejora o los síntomas persisten o empeoran, es necesario que consulte a su médico.

Efectos secundarios (molestias)

Esta medicina le puede causar ardor, comezón o irritación.

Instrucciones

1. Lávese bien las manos con agua y jabón antes y después de aplicar la medicina.
2. Lávese y séquese el área genital.
3. Abra el tubo (así). Mire, coloque la tapa al revés en el tubo para romper el sello.
4. Conecte el aplicador al tubo.
5. Oprima el tubo para llenar el aplicador con la crema.
6. Acuéstese boca arriba con las piernas separadas y dobladas o párese con los pies separados y las rodillas ligeramente dobladas.
7. Suavemente introduzca todo el aplicador dentro de la vagina.
8. Empuje el émbolo para depositar la crema dentro de la vagina.
9. Retire el aplicador y lávelo y enjuáguelo muy bien.
10. Si el aplicador es desechable, tírelo a la basura.

Consejos adicionales

1. Puede usar una toalla sanitaria mientras esté usando la medicina. No use tampones.
2. Puede usar la medicina también durante los días de la regla.
3. Si piensa que está embarazada, mejor vaya con su doctor.

Via de administración

Esta crema es sólo para uso vaginal.

Las preguntas fundamentales[2]

Srta. Ramos, le di muchas instrucciones. Me gustaría repasarlas con usted.

1. ¿Para qué es esta medicina?
   Esta medicina es para tratar la infección vaginal producida por un hongo.

2. ¿Cómo va a aplicar esta medicina?
   Es una crema que se aplica en la vagina. Voy a aplicarme la crema dentro de la vagina por las noches durante 3 días, al acostarme.

3. ¿Cuáles son los efectos secundarios?
   Esta medicina me puede causar ardor, comezón o irritación.

4. Quiero confirmar que no se me olvidó nada. Por favor, dígame cómo va a usar esta medicina.
   Sí, claro. Es una crema que se aplica en la vagina. Voy a aplicarme la crema dentro de la vagina durante 3 días al acostarme. Esta medicina me puede causar algo de ardor, comezón o irritación.

Señorita, que se sienta mejor pronto. Si siguen las molestias, vaya con su doctor.

Gracias por su consejo.

Gracias por su preferencia y que le vaya muy bien.

Audio dialogues

PHARMACIST: Good morning. I am Janet Harris, the pharmacist. How can I help you?

PATIENT: *It's a pleasure, Dr. Harris. Good morning. I am Ana Ramos, and I need for you to recommend to me (some) effective product . . . I have a lot of irritation in my . . . well, you know, . . . down there, that is (to say) in my private parts . . . in my vagina. I am very embarrassed, and I don't know what to use. I have a lot of itching.*

PHARMACIST: I'm sorry, Miss Ramos, but don't be embarrassed. This problem is very common. Let's see. First, I need to ask you some questions before I can recommend (to you) a product to treat the problem.

PATIENT: *Oh, I see. I understand.*

Questions[1]

1. What are your symptoms?
   I feel irritation, burning, lots of stinging.
   Do you have itching in the vaginal area?
   Oh, yes.
   Do you have discharge (fluid-like) or is there some discharge?
   Yes, I have a little discharge (fluid-like).
   Is it white or thick?
   Yes, it is whitish.
   Is there redness?
   Yes, I think so. Also, I feel swollen.
   Do you have irritation?
   Yes, the entire area is irritated.
   Does it (the genital area) hurt?
   Yes, some. I feel very uncomfortable.
   Have you noticed a bad odor in the discharge or from (in) your private parts?
   No, I don't think so.

2. Have you had other types of vaginal infections in the past?
   Yes, 3 years ago.

3. How long have you had the symptoms?
   Since the day before yesterday.

4. Are you taking medications or using a cream for the genital area?
   No, I am not using anything (nothing)

5. Are you using or taking some antibiotic?
   No, no medicine.

6. Are you pregnant or trying to get pregnant during these (next) days?
   No, I think that I am not pregnant and I am taking contraceptives to prevent (avoid) pregnancy.

Recommendations

Oh, good. I am going to recommend miconazole 4% cream. This medicine is for treating a vaginal infection caused by a fungus. It is a cream that one inserts vaginally. Insert the cream into the vagina for 3 days before going to bed. If you don't see an improvement or the symptoms persist or worsen, it is necessary for you to consult your doctor.

Side effects

This medicine may cause (you) burning, itching, or irritation.

Directions

1. Wash your hands well with water and soap before and after inserting the medicine.

2. Wash and dry the genital area.
3. Open the tube (like this). Look, place the cap backward in the tube to break seal.
4. Attach the applicator to the tube.
5. Squeeze the tube to fill applicator with cream.
6. Lie on your back with knees bent and open, or stand with your feet slightly apart and knees bent.
7. Gently insert the entire applicator into the vagina.
8. Push the plunger all the way to deposit cream into vagina.
9. Remove the applicator, and wash and rinse it very well.
10. If it is a disposable applicator, throw it away in the trash.

Other advice

1. You may use a sanitary pad while using the medicine. Do not use tampons.
2. You may also use the medicine during the days of your period.
3. If you think that you are pregnant, it is better that you see (go to) your doctor.

Administration route

This cream is for vaginal use only.

Prime questions[2]

Miss Ramos, I gave you a lot of instructions. I would like to review them with you.

1. What is the medication for?
   This medicine is to treat a vaginal infection caused by a fungus.

2. How are you going to apply the medication?
   It is a cream that one inserts vaginally. I will insert (into myself) the cream into the vagina in the evenings for 3 days, when (at) I go to sleep (lie down).

3. What are the side effects?
   This medicine may cause burning, itching, or irritation.

4. I want to make sure that I didn't forget anything. Please, tell me how you are going to use this medicine.
   Sure. It is a cream that one inserts into the vagina. I am going to insert the cream into my vagina for 3 days when (at) going to bed (lying down). This medicine may cause (me) burning, itching, or irritation.

Miss, may you feel better soon. If the problems continue, see (go with) your doctor.

Thank you for your advice.

Thank you for your patronage and may all go very well.

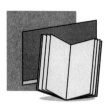

Lección 2   Supositorios rectales
Lesson 2   Rectal suppositories

This lesson does not include introductory questions. It focuses on directions for use of medication. For questions related to constipation, see chapter 4.

Recomendaciones

Esta medicina es un supositorio de bisacodyl de 10 mg. Es para tratar el estreñimiento.
Aplíquese 1 supositorio diariamente.

Efectos secundarios (molestias)

Los efectos secundarios son cólicos o diarrea.

Instrucciones[3]

1. Lávese las manos antes y después de usar la medicina.
2. Lávese y séquese el área rectal.
3. Quítele la envoltura al supositorio. Más específico: Con agua tibia, humedezca el supositorio dentro de su envoltura para suavizarlo.
4. Acuéstese de lado.
5. Use un dedo para empujar el supositorio dentro del recto.

Consejos adicionales

1. Refrigere el supositorio para endurecerlo si está demasiado blando.
2. Use papel sanitario o un dedal de hule para evitar el contacto con los dedos.

Vía de administración

Sólo para uso rectal

Las preguntas fundamentales[2]

1. ¿Para qué es esta medicina?
2. ¿Cómo va a aplicar esta medicina?
3. ¿Cuáles son los efectos secundarios?
4. Quiero confirmar que no se me olvidó nada. Por favor, dígame cómo va a usar esta medicina.

Recommendations

This medicine is a bisacodyl suppository 10 mg. It is for constipation.
Insert 1 suppository daily.

Side effects

The side effects are abdominal cramping or diarrhea.

Directions[3]

1. Wash your hands before and after using medicine.
2. Wash and dry the rectal area.
3. Remove the wrapper of the suppository. More specifically: With warm water, moisten (wet) the suppository inside its wrapper to soften it.
4. Lie down on your side.
5. Use a finger to push the suppository into the rectum.

Additional advice

1. Refrigerate the suppository to harden it if it is too soft.
2. Use toilet paper or a rubber finger cot to avoid contact with the fingers.

Administration route

For rectal use only

Prime questions[2]

1. What is this medication for?
2. How are you going to apply this medication?
3. What are the side effects?
4. I want to make sure that I didn't forget anything. Please, tell me how you are going to use this medication.

Diálogos para el audio

FARMACÉUTICO: Buenas noches. ¿En qué puedo ayudarle?

PACIENTE: *Buenas noches, ¿es usted el farmacéutico?*

FARMACÉUTICO: Sí efectivamente, soy el Dr. Gámez. Dígame.

PACIENTE: *Mire, es algo penoso pero hace 2 días que no puedo ir al baño. Estoy estreñido y me siento muy incómodo. Generalmente no acostumbro tomar laxantes ni tampoco uso supositorios. Pero mi estilo de vida en estas últimas semanas ha sido muy inestable. Es decir, no he comido bien. He tenido un alto nivel de estrés. No he dormido casi nada ni tampoco he hecho ejercicio. Y creo que por eso estoy estreñido. Necesito algo que me dé alivio rápido.*

FARMACÉUTICO: Entiendo. Claro que es mejor evitar el estreñimiento, pero hay unos medicamentos eficaces y seguros que le pueden servir.

Recomendaciones

Le voy a recomendar esta medicina. Es un supositorio de bisacodyl de 10 miligramos. Es un laxante que estimula el intestino. Aplíquese 1 supositorio diariamente. Dura de 15 minutos hasta 1 hora para funcionar.

Efectos secundarios (molestias)

Los efectos secundarios pueden ser cólicos o diarrea.

Instrucciones[3]

Para usar un supositorio:
1. Lávese las manos antes y después de usar la medicina.
2. Lávese y séquese el área rectal.
3. Quítele la envoltura al supositorio. Con agua tibia, puede humedecer el supositorio dentro de su envoltura para suavizarlo.
4. Acuéstese de lado.
5. Con un dedo empuje el supositorio dentro del recto.

Consejos adicionales

1. Refrigere el supositorio para endurecerlo si está demasiado blando.
2. Use papel sanitario o un dedal de hule para evitar el contacto con los dedos.

Vía de administración

El supositorio es sólo para uso rectal.

Las preguntas fundamentales[2]

Señor, le he dado muchas instrucciones.

1. Por favor, dígame ¿para qué es esta medicina?
   Esta medicina es un supositorio para aliviar el estreñimiento.

2. ¿Cómo va a usar esta medicina?
   Le quito la envoltura al supositorio. Me acuesto de lado. Con un dedo me aplico el supositorio.

3. ¿Cuáles son los efectos secundarios?
   Algunas de las molestias pueden ser cólicos o diarrea.

4. Quiero confirmar que no se me olvidó nada. Por favor, dígame cómo va a usar esta medicina.
   Sí, claro. Me acuesto de lado. Uso un dedo para empujar el supositorio dentro del recto. Me lavo bien las manos. Espero que me funcione rápido.

Sí. Muy bien. Que se sienta mejor.

Gracias por su ayuda, doctor.

Audio dialogues

PHARMACIST (MALE): Good evening. How can I help you?

PATIENT: *Good evening. Are you the pharmacist?*

PHARMACIST: Yes, I am Dr. Gámez. Tell me.

PATIENT: *Look, it is somewhat embarrassing, but I have not gone to the bathroom for 2 days. I am constipated, and I feel very uncomfortable. Generally, I am not used (accustomed) to taking laxatives, nor do I use suppositories. But my lifestyle these past few weeks has been very unstable. That is (to say), I have not eaten well. I have had a high level of stress. I haven't slept (almost) at all nor have I exercised. And I believe that's why (for this) I am constipated. I need something that works fast.*

PHARMACIST: I understand. Of course, it is better to avoid constipation, but there are some effective and safe medications that can help you.

Recommendations

I am going to recommend (to you) this medicine. It is a 10 milligram bisacodyl suppository. It is a laxative that stimulates the intestines. Insert (in yourself) 1 suppository daily. It can take (last) from 15 minutes to 1 hour to work (function).

Side effects

The side effects may be abdominal cramping or diarrhea.

Directions[3]

To use a suppository:
1. Wash your hands before and after using medicine.
2. Wash and dry your rectal area.
3. Remove the wrapper of the suppository. With warm water, you can moisten the suppository inside its wrapper to soften it.
4. Lie down on your side.
5. With a finger push the suppository into the rectum.

Additional advice

1. Refrigerate the suppository to harden it if it is too soft.
2. Use toilet paper or a rubber finger cot to avoid finger contact.

Administration route

The suppository is only for rectal use.

Prime questions[2]

Sir, I have given you a lot of instructions.
1. Please, tell me, what is this medication for?
   This medicine is a suppository to alleviate constipation.

2. How are you going to use this medication?
   I remove the wrapper of the suppository. I lie down on one side. With a finger, I insert (in myself) the suppository.

3. What are the side effects?
   Some side effects can be abdominal cramping or diarrhea.

4. I want to make sure that I didn't forget anything. Please, tell me how you are going to use this medication.
   Yes, of course. I lie down on one side. I use a finger to push the suppository inside the rectum. I will wash my hands well. I hope that it works fast.

Yes. Very good. May you feel better.

Thank you for your help, Doctor.

De la cultura / About the culture

1. In Latin America, women who are not sexually active often do not want to use medications or sanitary products (e.g., tampons) that have to be introduced into the vagina.

2. In some Latin American cultures, girls and young women commonly wash the vaginal area with an antiseptic and water. Women who are sexually active may use a douche for vaginal cleansing ("**lavados vaginales**").

3. The phrase "**estar embarazada**" means "to be pregnant," not "to be embarrassed." A person who is embarrassed would say "**me da pena**" or "**me da vergüenza**," meaning "it gives me embarrassment."

4. A doctor or pharmacist may use correct technical terms to talk about genitalia. Patients may even expect that the health care professional use a more technical term. However, patients may be embarrassed to use the technical words or may not be familiar with the technical terms. Rather, they will use nontechnical words to describe the body parts or use euphemisms. Pharmacy staff members should be sensitive about being private or talking in a quiet voice when counseling patients or directing them to personal products.

5. Many Spanish-speaking patients will use the term "**recto**" to refer to the "anus" because it sounds less offensive to them.

6. To ask if a woman is breastfeeding, the pharmacist may say, "**¿Está amamantado?**" or "**¿Le da pecho a su bebé?**" ("Are you breastfeeding?" or " Do you give breastmilk to your baby?")

Ejercicios / Exercises

I. Haga una pregunta para cada respuesta. (Write a question for each response.)

1. ¿_____?
   Tengo mucha comezón e irritación en mis partes privadas.

2. ¿_____?
   No, no he usado ninguna medicina, sólo me he dado lavados vaginales con un antiséptico.

3. ¿_____?
   No, nunca antes había tenido ninguna infección.

4. ¿_____?
   Tengo un desecho blanco que huele muy mal.

5. ¿_____?
   Voy a ponérmela con el aplicador dentro de la vagina.

II. Escriba una oración con las siguientes palabras. (Write a sentence using the following words.)

1. vagina / aplicador / crema

2. comezón / irritación / flujo

3. hongo / infección / medicamento

4. aplicar / supositorio / recto

5. refrigerar / medicamento / endurecer

III. Traduzca las siguientes expresiones al español. (Translate the following expressions into Spanish.)

1. Insert the medication using the applicator.

2. Lie down, face up.

3. Lie down to one side.

4. Stand with your knees slightly bent.

5. Deposit the cream using the applicator plunger.

6. You may use a sanitary napkin but not a tampon.

7. Remove the wrapper of the suppository.

IV. Relacione las palabras con su significado. (Match the words with their meaning.)

___ 1. la vulva	a. un supositorio hecho especialmente para usarse dentro de la vagina
___ 2. el supositorio rectal	b. el órgano genital femenino en el que se producen los óvulos
___ 3. el útero	c. una bolsa donde están los testículos
___ 4. el cervix	d. el órgano masculino externo que está sobre el escroto
___ 5. el óvulo vaginal	e. el período durante el cual se desarrolla el feto dentro del cuerpo de la madre
___ 6. el embarazo	f. los órganos que conectan los ovarios con la matriz
___ 7. el escroto	g. el órgano femenino donde se desarrolla el feto durante el embarazo
___ 8. el ovario	h. el cuello de la matriz
___ 9. las trompas de Falopio	i. el único órgano genital femenino externo
___10. el pene	j. un medicamento que se aplica por el recto

V. Busque en el Internet un sitio en español y escriba un párrafo sobre los siguientes temas.
(Look up an Internet site in Spanish and write a paragraph about the following topics.)

1. Los lavados vaginales

2. El prurito de los jockeys

3. El virus del papiloma humano (VPH)

4. Una infección de transmisión sexual

R E F E R E N C E S

1. Stack NM, Shimp LA. Vaginal and vulvovaginal disorders. In: Berardi RR, Kroon LA, McDermott JH, et al., eds. *Handbook of Nonprescription Drugs.* 15th ed. Washington, DC: American Pharmacists Association; 2006:135–54.
2. Gardner M, Boyce RW, Herrier RN. *Pharmacist–Patient Consultation Program PPCP-Unit I: An Interactive Approach to Verifying Patient Understanding.* New York: Pfizer Educational Services; 1991.
3. Curry CE Jr, Butler DM. Constipation. In: Berardi RR, Kroon LA, McDermott JH, et al., eds. *Handbook of Nonprescription Drugs.* 15th ed. Washington, DC: American Pharmacists Association; 2006:299–326.

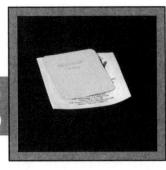

Parches, chicles y las tabletas sublinguales

Patches, gum, and sublingual tablets

Verbos / Verbs		Presente / Present tense			
		Yo	Él, ella, usted	Mandato	Ejemplos
colocar	to place	coloco	coloca	Coloque	*Coloque el chicle entre las mejillas y las encías.*
comenzar	to start, to begin	comienzo	comienza	Comience	*Cuando le comience el dolor, tome una tableta.*
contraer	to contract, to acquire a disease	contraigo	contrae	No contraiga	*Puede contraer cáncer si fuma.*
creer	to believe	creo	cree	Crea	*Creo que tengo una adicción muy fuerte a la nicotina.*
dejar (de)	to leave out, to stop	dejo (de)	deja (de)	Deje (de)	*Deje de fumar.*
mejorar(se)	to feel better	me mejoro	se mejora	Mejórese	*¡Que se mejore muy pronto!*
regresar	to return	regreso	regresa	Regrese	*El sabor a pimienta regresa en algunos minutos.*
reponer	to replace	repongo	repone	Reponga	*Reponga el parche cada semana.*
saber	to know	sé	sabe	Sepa	*¿Sabe las instrucciones?*

Sustantivos / Nouns

la adicción	addiction
el agrandamiento	enlargement
el apoyo	help, support
los bochornos	hot flashes
el chicle	gum (chewing)
la dependencia	dependency
el desvanecimiento	fainting
las encías	gums (in mouth)
el ensanchamiento de los senos	breast enlargement
el hambre	hunger
la histerectomía	hysterectomy
el hormigueo	tingling
la mascota	pet
las mejillas	cheeks
la menopausia	menopause
el parche	patch
la presión	pressure
el sabor a pimienta	peppery taste
los senos adoloridos	breast tenderness
la sensación	sensation
el sentimiento de soledad	loneliness
la toxicidad	toxicity
el vello	body hair

Otras expresiones / Other expressions

al mismo tiempo	at the same time
"el cambio de vida"	menopause (the change of life)
como de costumbre	usually
crear dependencia a...	to create dependency on...
dejar de fumar	quit smoking
demasiado(a)	too much
diariamente	daily
emotivo(a)	emotional
fuera del alcance	out of reach
otra vez	again
sensibilidad	sensitivity
síndrome de abstinencia	withdrawal
tener ganas	to feel like, to have the urge
todavía	still

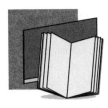

Lección 1   Parches de estrógeno
Lesson 1   Estrogen patch

Preguntas[1]
1. ¿Cuáles son sus síntomas? ¿Qué síntomas tiene?
   - ¿Tiene bochornos?
   - ¿Ha estado irritable últimamente?
   - ¿Tiene depresión? o ¿Está deprimida?
   - ¿Está más sentimental o emotiva de lo normal?
2. ¿Desde cuándo ha tenido estos síntomas?
3. ¿Está tomando medicamentos, hierbas o tés?
4. ¿Tiene la matriz o le hicieron una histerectomía?

Recomendaciones
Parche de estradiol 0.025 mg por día. Aplíqueselo cada semana.
1. Esta medicina contiene un tipo de estrógeno.
2. Es para controlar las molestias de la menopausia como los bochornos o la irritabilidad.
3. Aplíquese un parche nuevo cada semana.

Efectos secundarios (molestias)
1. Esta medicina le puede provocar hinchazón, dolor de cabeza, mareos, senos adoloridos, ensanchamiento (agrandamiento) de los senos o inflamación del vientre.
2. Es importante hablar con su doctor sobre los riesgos de contraer cáncer de seno o enfermedades del corazón.

Instrucciones
1. Lávese las manos antes y después de aplicarse el parche.
2. Aplíqueselo cada vez en un lugar diferente. La piel debe estar seca, limpia, y sin vello.
3. Debe aplicarse el parche en el vientre, los muslos o las asentaderas. No debe aplicárselo en los senos u otro lugar más arriba de la cintura.
4. Quite y reponga el parche al mismo tiempo cada semana.
5. Ponga el parche viejo en la envoltura original y tírelo a la basura.

Etiqueta de los productos
Manténgalo fuera del alcance de los niños y las mascotas.

Las preguntas fundamentales[2]
1. ¿Para qué es esta medicina?
2. ¿Cómo va a aplicar esta medicina?
3. ¿Cuáles son los efectos secundarios?
4. Quiero confirmar que no olvidé nada. Ahora ¿me puede explicar cómo va a usar esta medicina?

Questions[1]

1. What are your symptoms? What symptoms to you have?
   - Do you have hot flashes?
   - Have you been irritable lately?
   - Do you have depression? Or are you depressed?
   - Do you feel more emotional than usual?
2. How long have you had these symptoms?
3. Are you taking any medicine, herbs, or teas?
4. Do you still have your uterus, or have you had a hysterectomy?

Recommendations

Estradiol patches 0.025 mg/day. Apply (to yourself) each week.

1. This medicine contains a type of estrogen.
2. It is prescribed to prevent the effects of menopause such as hot flashes or irritability.
3. Apply (to yourself) a new patch each week.

Side effects

1. This medication may cause swelling, headache, dizziness, breast tenderness, breast enlargement, or bloating.
2. It is important to talk with your doctor about the risks of getting breast cancer or heart disease.

Directions

1. Wash your hands before and after applying the patch.
2. Apply (to yourself) each time to a different place. The skin must be dry, clean, and hairless.
3. You should apply (to yourself) the patch on the abdomen, thighs, or buttocks. Do not apply over the breasts or anywhere above the waistline.
4. Remove and replace the patch at the same time each week.
5. Put the old patch in the original wrapper and throw it in the trash.

Product labeling

Keep out of the reach of children and pets.

Prime questions[2]

1. What is this medication for?
2. How are you going to apply this medication?
3. What are the side effects?
4. I want to make sure I didn't forget anything. Now, can you explain to me how you are going to use this medicine?

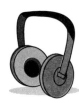

Diálogos para el audio

FARMACÉUTICO: Buenos días. Soy el Dr. Cohen. ¿En qué le puedo servir?

PACIENTE: *Buenos días, Doctor. Yo soy Guillermina Flores. Últimamente me he sentido muy mal. Creo que es por los cambios de la menopausia. Fui a ver al doctor y me dio esta receta para un parche. Pero no entendí realmente cuáles son los síntomas de la menopausia, ni cómo usar la medicina y por lo tanto, no me he puesto el parche todavía.*

FARMACÉUTICO: Mucho gusto, Sra. Flores. Bueno, le voy a hacer algunas preguntas, y luego le explico cómo usar el medicamento.

Preguntas[1]

1. ¿Cuáles son sus síntomas?
   Me siento deprimida y con falta de energía.

   ¿Tiene bochornos?
   Sí, tengo muchos bochornos y sudo tanto por las noches que me tengo que levantar a cambiarme la ropa de dormir.

   ¿Ha estado irritable últimamente?
   Muy irritable. Mi esposo y mis hijos dicen que estoy de mal humor.

   ¿Tiene depresión?
   Me siento un poco triste. Me dan muchas ganas de llorar.

   ¿Está más sentimental o emotiva de lo normal?
   Mucho más de lo normal y lloro muy seguido. Yo antes no era así.

2. ¿Desde cuándo ha tenido estos síntomas?
   Me empezaron hace más o menos 3 meses. Al principio, pensé que era algo pasajero, pero se me han agravado muchísimo todos esos malestares. Además todo el tiempo me siento cansada.

3. ¿Está tomando medicamentos, hierbas o tés?
   No, actualmente no estoy tomando nada.

4. ¿Tiene la matriz o le hicieron una histerectomía?
   Sí, hace un mes que me quitaron la matriz y los ovarios. Desde entonces, me he sentido peor, pero no quería quejarme ni comprar la medicina.

Bueno, probablemente usted tiene un nivel bajo de hormonas debido a la menopausia provocada por la cirugía. Yo creo que esto le está causando los síntomas y malestares.

Recomendaciones

Su doctor le recetó esta medicina que es un parche de estradiol de 0.025 mg por día. Esta medicina contiene un tipo de estrógeno. Es para controlar las molestias de la menopausia como los bochornos y la irritabilidad. Aplíquese un parche nuevo cada semana.

Efectos secundarios (molestias)

Esta medicina le puede provocar hinchazón, dolor de cabeza, mareos, senos adoloridos, agrandamiento de los senos o inflamación del vientre. Son molestias similares a las que sentía cuando tenía la regla.

Es importante hablar con su doctor sobre los riesgos de contraer cáncer de seno o enfermedades del corazón.

Ah, gracias por explicarme porqué tengo estas molestias. Ahora voy a poder ponerme el parche con más confianza.

Bueno, pero todavía quiero explicarle cómo va a usar este parche.

Instrucciones

1. Lávese las manos antes y después de aplicarse el parche.
2. Aplíqueselo en un lugar diferente cada vez. La piel debe estar seca, limpia, y sin vello.
3. Debe aplicarse el parche en el vientre, los muslos o las asentaderas. No debe aplicárselo en los senos u otro lugar más arriba de la cintura.
4. Quítese el parche y repóngalo al mismo tiempo cada semana.
5. Ponga el parche viejo en la envoltura original y tírelo a la basura.

Etiqueta de los productos

Manténgalo fuera del alcance de los niños y las mascotas.

Las preguntas fundamentales[2]

1. ¿Para qué es esta medicina?
   Para aliviar los malestares de la menopausia.

2. ¿Cómo va a aplicarse esta medicina?
   Me voy a poner el parche cada semana en un lugar diferente cada vez . . . en las asentaderas, los muslos o el vientre.

3. ¿Cuáles son los efectos secundarios?
   Pueden provocarme dolor de cabeza, hinchazón de los senos o inflamación abdominal.

4. Quiero confirmar que no olvidé nada. Ahora ¿me puede explicar cómo va a usar esta medicina?
   Voy a aplicarme un parche cada semana. Siempre hay que cambiarlo el mismo día de la semana.

Muy bien. Espero que se sienta mejor.

Gracias, Dr. Cohen. Que tenga buen día.

Audio dialogues

PHARMACIST: Good morning. I am Dr. Cohen. How can I help you?

PATIENT: *Good morning, doctor. I am Guillermina Flores. Lately, I have felt really bad. I think that it is because of the changes of menopause. I went to see the doctor, and he gave me this prescription for a patch. But I didn't really understand what are the symptoms of menopause or how to use the medicine, and for this reason, I have not put the patch (on me) yet.*

PHARMACIST: Pleased to meet you, Mrs. Flores, Well, I am going to ask you some questions, and later I (will) explain to you how to use the medication.

Questions[1]

1. What are your symptoms?
   I feel depressed and (with) a lack of energy.

   Do you have hot flashes?
   Yes, I have a lot of hot flashes, and I sweat so much at night that I have to get up and change my night clothes.

   Have you been irritable lately?
   Very irritable. My husband and my children say that I am in a bad mood.

   Do you have depression?
   I feel a little sad. I really feel like crying.

   Are you more sensitive or emotional than usual?
   Much more than normal, and I cry very often. Before I wasn't like this.

2. How long have you had these symptoms?
   They began about (more or less) 3 months ago. At the beginning, I thought that it was something temporary, but all of these discomforts have gotten much worse for me. Besides, I feel tired all of the time.

3. Are you taking medications, herbs, or teas?
   No, really I am not taking anything (nothing).

4. Do you have your uterus, or have you had (did they make you) a hysterectomy?
   Yes, one month ago they took out my uterus and ovaries. Since then, I have felt worse, but I did not want to complain (myself) or (nor) buy medicine.

Well, probably you have a low hormone level secondary to menopause provoked by the surgery. I think that this is causing you all of the symptoms and discomforts.

Recommendations

Your doctor prescribed for you a medicine that is a patch of estradiol 0.025 mg per day. This medicine contains a type of estrogen. It is for controlling the side effects of menopause like hot flashes and irritability. Apply (to yourself) a new patch each week.

Side effects

This medicine can cause you swelling, headache, dizziness, breast tenderness, breast enlargement, or bloating. These effects are similar to how you felt when you had periods.

It is important to talk with your doctor about the risks of getting (contracting) breast cancer or heart disease.

Oh, thank you for explaining to me why I have these side effects. Now I am going to be able to put the patch on (myself) with more confidence.

Very well, but I still want to explain to you how to use this patch.

Instructions

1. Wash your hand before and after applying (to yourself) the patch.
2. Apply it to (yourself) in a different place each time. The skin must be dry, clean, and without (body) hair.
3. You must apply the patch (to yourself) on the abdomen, thighs, or buttocks. Do not apply it (to yourself) on the breasts or another place (more) above the waist.
4. Remove the patch and replace it at the same time each week.
5. Put the old patch in the original wrapper and throw it in the trash.

Product labeling

Keep it out of the reach of children and pets.

Prime questions[2]

1. What is this medicine for?
   For the discomforts of menopause.

2. How are you going to apply this medicine?
   I am going to put the patch on (myself) each week in a different place each time . . . on the buttocks, thighs, or abdomen.

3. What are the side effects?
   They can give me a headache, breast swelling, or bloating.

4. I want to confirm that I didn't forget anything. Now, can you explain to me how you are going to use the medicine?
   I am going to apply a patch (to myself) each week. Always it has to be changed on the same day of the week.

Very well. I hope that you feel better.

Thank you, Dr. Cohen. May you have a good day.

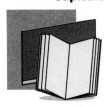

Lección 2 Chicles de nicotina
Lesson 2 Nicotine gum

Toxicidad de la nicotina	Síndrome de abstinencia
náusea	demasiada hambre
vómito	irritabilidad
diarrea	sentimiento de soledad
dolor de estómago	cansancio
confusión	depresión

Preguntas[3]

1. ¿Desde cuándo fuma?
2. ¿Cuántos cigarrillos fuma al día?
3. ¿Ha tratado de dejar de fumar antes?
4. ¿Por qué quiere dejar de fumar?
5. ¿Tiene apoyo para dejar de fumar?

Recomendaciones

Nicotina 2 mg

Voy a recomendarle un chicle de nicotina de 2 mg.
Puede usarlo cuando sienta ganas de fumar.
Esta medicina le va a ayudar a tener menos síntomas del síndrome de abstinencia.

Efectos secundarios (molestias)

Puede causar náusea, diarrea, malestar estomacal, sabor a pimienta, dolor de cabeza e hipo.

Instrucciones

1. Deje de fumar.
2. Mastique el chicle de una a dos veces. Va a sentir un hormigueo en la boca o un sabor a pimienta.
3. Coloque (ponga) el chicle entre las encías y las mejillas por 1 minuto.
4. Mastique el chicle otra vez hasta que el sabor o las sensaciones regresen.
5. Puede masticarlo durante 30 minutos.

Consejos adicionales

1. No fume mientras esté masticando el chicle de nicotina.
2. No se trague el chicle.
3. Evite los productos ácidos como los refrescos, el café, los jugos o las comidas picantes. Si los bebe o los come, enjuáguese la boca antes de masticar el chicle.
4. No use más de 24 chicles en un sólo día.

Etiqueta de los productos

Manténgase fuera del alcance de los niños.

Las preguntas fundamentales[2]

1. ¿Para qué es esta medicina?
2. ¿Cómo va a usar esta medicina?
3. ¿Cuáles son los efectos secundarios?
4. Quiero confirmar que no se me olvidó nada. Por favor, dígame cómo va a usar esta medicina.

Nicotine toxicity	Withdrawal symptoms
nausea	a lot of hunger
vomiting	irritability
diarrhea	loneliness
abdominal pain	fatigue
confusion	depression

Questions[3]

1. How long (Since when) have you smoked?
2. How many cigarettes do you smoke a day?
3. Have you tried to quit smoking before?
4. Why do you want to quit smoking?
5. Do you have support to quit smoking?

Recommendations

Nicotine 2 mg

I am going to recommend to you a nicotine gum 2 mg.
You can use it when you feel the urge to smoke.
This medicine is going to help you have fewer withdrawal symptoms.

Side effects

It may cause nausea, diarrhea, upset stomach, peppery taste, headache, and hiccups.

Directions

1. Stop smoking.
2. Chew the gum one to two times. You will feel a tingling (like ants) in your mouth or a peppery taste.
3. Place (put) the gum (chewing) between the gums (of your mouth) and the cheek for about 1 minute.
4. Chew the gum again until the peppery taste or sensations return.
5. You may chew it for about 30 minutes.

Additional advice

1. Do not smoke while chewing the nicotine gum.
2. Do not swallow the gum.
3. Avoid acidic products like soft drinks, coffee, juice, or spicy food. If you drink or eat them, rinse out your mouth before chewing the gum.
4. Do not use more than 24 pieces each day.

Product labeling

Keep out of reach of children.

Prime questions[2]

1. What is this medication for?
2. How are you going to use this medication?
3. What are the side effects?
4. I want to make sure I didn't forget anything. Please tell me how you are going to use this medicine.

Diálogos para el audio

FARMACÉUTICA: Buenos días. Soy la Dra. Karen Baker y soy su farmacéutica. ¿En qué le puedo ayudar?

PACIENTE: *Buenos días, doctora. Yo soy Abel Mendoza. Sabe que estoy tratando de dejar de fumar y quisiera saber si hay alguna medicina o tratamiento que me pueda ayudar. Hace 2 días dejé de fumar y ahora me siento muy mal y muy irritable.*

FARMACÉUTICA: Probablemente usted tiene los síntomas del síndrome de abstinencia. Su cuerpo está acostumbrado a la nicotina, y si deja de fumar, a su cuerpo le hace falta esta sustancia. Algunos síntomas del síndrome de abstinencia son sentir demasiada hambre, irritabilidad, sentimiento de soledad, cansancio o depresión. Me gustaría hacerle algunas preguntas.

Preguntas[3]

1. ¿Desde cuándo fuma?
   Desde hace 20 años. Empecé a fumar cuando tenía 15 años.

2. ¿Cuántos cigarrillos fuma al día?
   Fumo más o menos 10 cigarrillos diarios.

3. ¿Ha tratado de dejar de fumar antes?
   Sí, muchas veces, pero sin éxito.

4. ¿Por qué quiere dejar de fumar?
   Porque uno de mis hijos tiene asma y le hace daño el humo.

5. ¿Tiene apoyo para dejar de fumar?
   Pues, sí. Mis hijos me van a apoyar.

Recomendaciones

Bueno. Voy a recomendarle un chicle de nicotina de 2 mg. Puede usarlo cuando tenga ganas de fumar. Esta medicina le va a ayudar a tener menos síntomas del síndrome de abstinencia.

Efectos secundarios (molestias)

Puede causarle náusea, diarrea, malestar estomacal, sabor a pimienta, dolor de cabeza e hipo.

Instrucciones

Antes de usar esta medicina . . .
1. Deje de fumar.
2. Mastique el chicle de una a dos veces. Va a sentir un hormigueo en la boca o un sabor a pimienta.
3. Coloque el chicle entre las encías y las mejillas por 1 minuto.
4. Mastíquelo otra vez hasta que el sabor o las sensaciones regresen.
5. Puede masticarlo durante 30 minutos.

Consejos adicionales

1. Sobre todo, no fume mientras esté masticando el chicle de nicotina.

2. No se trague el chicle.
3. Evite productos ácidos como los refrescos, café, jugo o comidas picantes. Si los bebe o los come, enjuáguese la boca antes de masticar el chicle.
4. No use más de 24 chicles en un sólo día.

Etiqueta de los productos

Manténgalos fuera del alcance de los niños.

Las preguntas fundamentales[2]

Quiero confirmar que le expliqué bien. Dígame . . .
1. ¿Para qué es esta medicina?
   Es para los malestares que tengo por dejar de fumar.

2. ¿Cómo va a usar esta medicina?
   Voy a masticar un chicle de una a dos veces. Voy a sentir una sensación como un hormigueo en la boca o un sabor a pimienta. Lo voy a colocar entre las encías y las mejillas por un minuto. Lo mastico otra vez hasta que el sabor o las sensaciones regresen. Puedo masticarlo durante 30 minutos.

3. ¿Cuáles son los efectos secundarios?
   Me puede provocar náusea, diarrea, malestar estomacal, dolor de cabeza o hipo.

4. Quiero confirmar que no se me olvidó nada. Por favor, dígame cómo va a usar esta medicina.
   No voy a masticar los chicles como chicles regulares. Tengo que masticar un chicle de una a dos veces y después colocarlo entre las encías y las mejillas. Luego, voy a masticarlo otra vez cuando haya pasado la sensación de hormigueo.

Muy bien. Espero que los chicles le ayuden a dejar de fumar. Ojalá que se sienta mejor. Si necesita más ayuda, por favor regrese a la farmacia o llámenos.

Muchas gracias por su ayuda, doctora. Hasta luego.

Que le vaya bien.

Audio dialogues

PHARMACIST: Good morning. I am Dr. Karen Baker, and I am your pharmacist. How can I help you?

PATIENT: *Good morning, doctor. I am Abel Mendoza. You know that I am trying to quit (leave) smoking, and I would like to know if there is some medicine that can help me. It has been 2 days since I quit (left) smoking, and now I feel (myself) very bad and very irritable.*

PHARMACIST: Probably you have withdrawal symptoms. Your body is accustomed to the nicotine, and if you quit (leave) smoking, your body needs (has a lack of) this substance. Some withdrawal symptoms are to feel a lot of hunger, irritability, loneliness, tiredness, or depression. I would like to ask (make) you some questions.

Questions[3]

1. How long (Since when) have you smoked?
   For 20 years. I began to smoke when I was (had) 15 years (old).

2. How many cigarettes do you smoke a day?
   I smoke more or less 10 cigarettes daily.

3. Have you tried to quit (leave) smoking before?
   Yes, many times, but without success.

4. Why do you want to quit (leave) smoking?
   Because one of my children has asthma, and the smoke causes him harm.

5. Do you have support to quit (leave) smoking?
   Well, yes. My children are going to support me.

Recommendations

Good. I am going to recommend to you a 2 mg nicotine gum. You can use it when you have the urge to smoke. This medicine is going to help you have fewer withdrawal symptoms.

Side effects

It can cause you nausea, diarrhea, stomach discomfort, peppery taste, headache, and hiccups.

Directions

Before using this medicine . . .
1. Stop smoking.
2. Chew the gum one or two times. You will feel a tingling (like ants) in your mouth or a peppery taste.
3. Place (put) the (chewing) gum between (your) gums and the cheeks for about 1 minute.
4. Chew the gum again until the peppery taste or sensations return.
5. You may chew it for about 30 minutes.

Additional advice

1. Above all, do not smoke while chewing the nicotine gum.
2. Do not swallow the gum.

3. Avoid acidic products like soft drinks, coffee, juice, or spicy food. If you drink or eat them, rinse out your mouth before chewing the gum.
4. Do not use more than 24 pieces each day.

Product labeling

Keep out of reach of children.

Prime questions[2]

I want to confirm that I explained (to you) well. Tell me . . .
1. What is this medication for?
   It is for the discomforts that I have because of quitting (leaving) smoking.

2. How are you going to use this medication?
   I am going to chew the gum one to two times. I am going to feel a tingling sensation (like an ant) in the mouth or a peppery taste. I am going to place it between the gums and cheeks for a minute. I chew it again until the taste or sensations return. I can chew it for (during) 30 minutes.

3. What are the side effects?
   It can cause me nausea, diarrhea, stomach discomfort, peppery taste, headache, or hiccups.

4. I want to make sure I didn't forget anything. Please tell me how you are going to use this medicine.
   I am not going to chew the gum(s) like regular chewing gum(s). I have to chew a piece one or two times and then place it between the gums and the cheeks. Later, I am going to chew it again when the tingling sensation (of ants) has passed.

Very well. I hope that the gum(s) help you quit (leave) smoking. I hope that you feel better. If you need more help, please return to the pharmacy or call us.

Many thanks for your help, doctor. Until later.

May it go well for you.

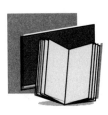

Lección 3 Nitroglicerina sublingual
Lesson 3 Sublingual nitroglycerin

Recomendaciones[1]

Nitroglicerina 0.4 mg

El doctor le recetó nitroglicerina de 0.4 mg.
Póngase 1 tableta debajo de la lengua cuando comience a sentir dolor en el pecho.
Puede hacerlo hasta dos veces más.
Si no se siente mejor, llame a su doctor o al 911.

Instrucciones

1. Si siente dolor en el pecho, póngase 1 tableta debajo de la lengua.
2. Espere 5 minutos.
3. Si no se siente mejor, póngase otra tableta.
4. Espere 5 minutos.
5. Puede ponerse hasta 1 tableta más. O sea, puede ponerse hasta 3 tabletas en total.
6. Si no se siente mejor después de 15 minutos máximo, llame inmediatamente al 911.

Efectos secundarios (molestias)

Esta medicina le podría provocar dolor de cabeza, mareos, desvanecimiento o presión baja.

Etiqueta de los productos

Manténgalo en un lugar seco y oscuro.

Las preguntas fundamentales[2]

1. ¿Para qué es esta medicina?
2. ¿Cómo va a usar esta medicina?
3. ¿Cuáles son los efectos secundarios?
4. Quiero confirmar que no se me olvidó nada. Por favor, dígame cómo va a usar esta medicina.

Recommendations[1]

Nitroglycerin 0.4 mg

The doctor prescribed you nitroglycerin 0.4 mg.
Put 1 tablet under your tongue when you start feeling a chest pain.
You may repeat it two more times.
If you don't feel better, call your doctor or 911.

Directions

1. If you feel chest pain, place 1 tablet under your tongue.
2. Wait 5 minutes.
3. If you do not feel better, take (place yourself) another tablet.
4. Wait 5 minutes.
5. You can take (place yourself) up to 1 more tablet. That is, you can take (place yourself) up to 3 tablets total.
6. If you do not feel better after at most 15 minutes, call 911 immediately.

Side effects

This medicine may cause headache, dizziness, fainting, or low blood pressure.

Product labeling

Keep in a dry, dark place.

Prime questions[2]

1. What is this medication for?
2. How are you going to use this medication?
3. What are the side effects?
4. I want to make sure I didn't forget anything. Please tell me how you are going to use this medicine.

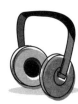

Diálogos para el audio

FARMACÉUTICA: Buenos días. Soy la Dra. Juanita Ramírez y soy su farmacéutica. ¿Cómo le puedo ayudar?

PACIENTE: *Buenos días, doctora. Pues traigo esta receta que me dio mi doctor para el corazón.*

FARMACÉUTICA: Muy bien, déjeme ver qué le recetaron.

Recomendaciones[1]

La medicina es nitroglicerina de 0.4 mg.
Póngase 1 tableta debajo de la lengua cuando comience a sentir dolor en el pecho.
Puede hacerlo hasta dos veces más.
Si no se siente mejor, llame a su doctor o al 911.

Ah, ¿es todo?

No, le quiero dar instrucciones adicionales para usar la medicina.

Instrucciones

1. Si siente dolor en el pecho, póngase 1 tableta debajo de la lengua.
2. Espere 5 minutos.
3. Si no se siente mejor, póngase otra tableta.
4. Espere 5 minutos.
5. Puede repetir una vez más. O sea, puede ponerse hasta 3 tabletas.
6. Pero, si no se siente mejor después de 15 minutos máximo, llame inmediatamente al 911.

Efectos secundarios (molestias)

Esta medicina le podría provocar dolor de cabeza, mareos, desvanecimiento o presión baja.

Etiqueta de los productos

Manténgalo en un lugar seco y oscuro.

Las preguntas fundamentales[2]

1. ¿Para qué es esta medicina?
   Es para el corazón, cuando me duela el pecho.

2. ¿Cómo va a usar esta medicina?
   Me voy a poner la tableta debajo de la lengua cuando sienta el dolor en el pecho.

3. ¿Cuáles son los efectos secundarios?
   Me puede provocar dolor de cabeza, mareos o desvanecimiento o que se me baje la presión.

4. Quiero confirmar que no se me olvidó nada. Por favor, repita cómo va a usar esta medicina.
   Me voy a poner 1 tableta debajo de la lengua y puedo ponerme hasta 3 tabletas, pero si no se me quita el dolor tengo que llamar al 911.

Creo que entendió muy bien las instrucciones. Espero que se sienta mejor.

Gracias, doctora. Yo también espero que la medicina me alivie el dolor.

Audio dialogues

PHARMACIST: Good morning. I am Dr. Juanita Ramirez, and I am your pharmacist. How can I help you?

PATIENT: *Good morning, Doctor. Well, I bring this prescription that my doctor gave me for my heart.*

PHARMACIST: Very well, let me see what they prescribed for you.

Recommendations[1]

The medicine is nitroglycerin 0.4 mg.

Put 1 tablet under your tongue when you start feeling a chest pain.

You may repeat it two more times.

If you don't feel better, call your doctor or 911.

Ah, is that all?

No, I want to give you additional directions for using the medicine.

Directions

1. If you feel chest pain, place 1 tablet under your tongue.
2. Wait 5 minutes.
3. If you do not feel better, take (place on yourself) another tablet.
4. Wait 5 minutes.
5. You can repeat (this) one more time. That is, you can take (place yourself) up to 3 tablets.
6. But, if you do not feel better after 15 minutes maximum, call 911 immediately.

Side effects

This medicine may cause you headache, dizziness, fainting, or low blood pressure.

Product labeling

Keep it in a dry, dark place.

Prime questions[2]

1. What is this medication for?
   It is for the heart, when my chest hurts me.

2. How are you going to use this medication?
   I am going to put (myself) a tablet under the tongue when I feel pain in the chest.

3. What are the side effects?
   It can cause me headache, dizziness, or fainting or lower my blood pressure.

4. I want to make sure I didn't forget anything. Please repeat how you are going to use this medicine.
   I am going to put (myself) 1 tablet under the tongue, and I can take up to 3 tablets, but if the pain doesn't go away, I have to call 911.

I think that you understood very well the instructions. I hope that you feel better.

Thank you, Doctor. I also hope that the medicine improves (alleviates) the pain.

De la cultura / About the culture

1. Some Spanish-speaking patients will not know the technical term "menopausia." Instead, they may use the phrase "el cambio de vida" or "the change of life" to talk about the changes in mood and in life that occur at menopause. If the pharmacist notices that a patient does not seem to understand the term "menopausia," he or she may find it helpful to say "el cambio de vida."

2. In most of Latin America, the habit of smoking has traditionally been acceptable. In general, people have been able to smoke in public places. However, public policy in Latin America is changing, and the prohibition of smoking in public buildings is becoming more common.

3. Several different words are used for cigarettes, including "cigarrillo," "cigarro," or "cigarrito." However, sometimes "cigarro" also refers to cigars, as does the word "puro."

4. In Latin America, chewing gum is considered somewhat rude. You would only chew gum at home, in your car, or in very informal situations. It is considered very rude to chew gum at work if you are attending a meeting or have to talk with other people. Still, many people chew gum after meals if they do not have a chance to brush their teeth, to clean them and to clear their breath. This practice is considered polite.

5. In Hispanic cultures, complementary alternative medicine (e.g., herbal products) is often used to treat many illnesses and symptoms. Traditional healers are also sometimes consulted (e.g., curanderos, santeros, sobadores, or espiritistas) to treat illnesses. Some common folk illnesses include "empacho," an illness of the stomach; "susto," a type of fright that can induce an illness; and "mal de ojo," an illness caused by a jealous or negative intention of one person to another ("evil eye").[4]

Ejercicios / Exercises

I. Escriba una pregunta para cada respuesta. (Write a question for each answer.)

1. _____
   Tengo muchos malestares a causa del "el cambio de vida."

2. _____
   Todavía tengo la matriz, pero creo que ya estoy en la menopausia.

3. _____
   Hay unos medicamentos muy buenos, por ejemplo el chicle de nicotina.

4. _____
   No sé cuántas veces debo tomar esta tableta, ni para qué sirve.

5. _____
   Creo que voy a sentir un hormigueo en la boca y un sabor a pimienta.

II. Escriba una oración con las siguientes palabras. (Write a sentence with the following words.)

1. la menopausia / los bochornos / la irritabilidad

2. la histerectomía / el parche / la medicina

3. los efectos secundarios / el aumento de peso / la inflamación del vientre

4. el chicle / masticar / 30 minutos

5. debajo de la lengua / ponerse

III. Relacione las palabras con su significado. (Match the words with their meaning.)

1. _____ la menopausia

2. _____ el síndrome de abstinencia

3. _____ la tableta sublingual

4. _____ los bochornos

5. _____ el hormigueo

6. _____ la adicción

7. _____ la toxicidad

8. _____ el malestar

9. _____ la histerectomía

a. quitar la matriz con una cirugía

b. sensación en la boca u otra parte del cuerpo en la que se siente como si tuviera hormigas caminando

c. efectos secundarios muy adversos que causan algunos medicamentos

d. síntomas del paciente debido a una enfermedad que son desagradables o dolorosas.

e. el hábito de usar algunas substancias químicas para cambiar el estado de ánimo

f. medicamento en tabletas que se pone debajo de la lengua

g. los malestares que padece un paciente cuando deja de usar una substancia a la que es adicto

h. calor súbito que experimentan las mujeres en la parte superior del cuerpo debido a la menopausia

i. cambio bioquímico del cuerpo de la mujer en el cual deja de ser fértil

IV. Escriba la forma correcta de los verbos. (Write the correct form of the verbs.)

1. (dejar, usar) Para _____ la adicción al tabaco (tabaquismo) _____ los chicles de nicotina. Es un tratamiento efectivo y seguro.

2. (creer, tener) ¿Usted _____ que ya _____ la menopausia?

3. (colocar) _____ el chicle entre las encías y las mejillas por un minuto.

4. (estar, tener, estar) Algunas mujeres que _____ en la edad madura, _____ muchas molestias debido a la menopausia y _____ muy irritables.

V. Busque en el Internet un sitio en español y escriba un párrafo sobre uno de los siguientes temas. (Look up an Internet site in Spanish and write a paragraph about one of the following themes.)

1. la menopausia

2. la adicción al tabaco (tabaquismo)

3. dolor de pecho

REFERENCES

1. Lacy CF, Armstrong LL, Goldman MP, Lance LL. *Drug Information Handbook.* 17th ed. Hudson, Ohio: Lexi-Comp; 2005.
2. Gardner M, Boyce RW, Herrier RN. *Pharmacist–Patient Consultation Program PPCP-Unit I: An Interactive Approach to Verifying Patient Understanding.* New York: Pfizer Educational Services; 1991.
3. Hudmon KS, Kroon LA, Corelli RL. Smoking cessation. In: Berardi RR, Kroon LA, McDermott JH, et al., eds. *Handbook of Nonprescription Drugs.* 15th ed. Washington, DC: American Pharmacists Association; 2006:1021–44.
4. National Alliance for Hispanic Health. *Delivering Health Care to Hispanics: A Manual for Providers.* 4th ed. Washington, DC: Estrella Press; 2007.

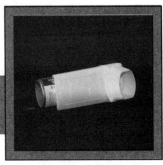

Inhaladores orales y nasales
Oral and nasal inhalers

Verbos / Verbs		Presente / Present tense			
		Yo	Él, ella, usted	Mandato	Ejemplo
empeorar	to worsen	empeoro	empeora	No empeore	*¿Qué le **empeora** el asma?*
escupir	to spit	escupo	escupe	Escupa	*Haga buches con la medicina y **escupa.***
exhalar	to exhale	exhalo	exhala	Exhale	***Exhale** lentamente.*
faltar	to be lacking	falto	falta	Falte	*Me **falta** el aliento muy seguido.*
inhalar	to inhale	inhalo	inhala	Inhale	***Inhale** profundamente.*
inspirar	to inhale, to inspire	inspiro	inspira	Inspire	***Inspire** y contenga la respiración.*
mostrar	to show	muestro	muestra	Muestre(me)	***Muéstreme** cómo usar el inhalador.*
respirar	to breathe	respiro	respira	Respire	***Respire** normalmente.*
sonar(se)	to blow one's nose	me sueno	se suena	Suénese	***Suénese** la nariz.*
soplar	to blow out	soplo	sopla	Sople	***Sople** despacio.*

Sustantivos / Nouns

el aparato	apparatus, device
el atomizador	spray
el barril	barrel (of inhaler)
el dispositivo	device
la emergencia	emergency
el exterior	exterior
la inhalación	inhalation, puff
el principio	the beginning
el rocío	sprinkle, aerosol
la sien	temple
el silbido	wheezing

El ambiente / Environment

los ácaros del polvo	dust mites
el(los) alérgeno(s)	allergen(s)
la caspa animal	animal dander
la espora	spore
la fiebre de heno	hay fever

el humo	smoke
el humo de segunda mano	secondhand smoke
el medio ambiente	environment
el moho	mold, mildew
el perfume	perfume
la planta	plant
el polen	pollen
el polvo	dust

Las estaciones / Seasons

el invierno	winter
el otoño	autumn/fall
la primavera	spring
el verano	summer

Otras expresiones / Other expressions

el algodoncillo (slang)	oral thrush (cotton-like)
el ataque de asma	asthma attack
contener la respiración	hold the breath

la enfermedad crónica	chronic illness
la falta de aliento	shortness of breath
haga buches	swish
el hongo de la boca	fungus of the mouth
la infección bucal por hongos	oral thrush
lentamente	slowly
la opresión en el pecho	chest tightness
el paciente asmático	asthmatic patient
por dentro	inside
profundo(a)	deep
los tubos de extensión	"spacers"
las vías respiratorias	airway passages

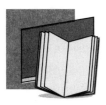

Lección 1 Inhalador oral
Lesson 1 Oral inhaler

Preguntas con respecto al asma[1]
1. ¿En qué época del año le empeora el asma? ¿Durante la primavera, el verano, el otoño o el invierno?
2. Por favor, dígame con qué se siente peor.
3. ¿Tiene alergias a las plantas, por ejemplo? ¿A otras cosas?
4. ¿Tiene tos, flema, falta de aliento, un silbido al respirar u opresión en el pecho?

Recomendaciones
Inhalador de albuterol (para el asma)
Haga de 1 a 2 inhalaciones cada 4 a 6 horas si es necesario para la falta de aliento (o en caso de emergencia).

Instrucciones
1. Quite la tapa.
2. Agite el inhalador. (Agítelo bien.)
3. Sople (exhale) lentamente.
4. Hay dos maneras para usar su inhalador:
    a. Introduzca el inhalador en la boca. Cierre la boca sobre el inhalador.
    b. Coloque el inhalador de 1 a 2 pulgadas (de 2 a 5 centímetros) de la boca abierta.
5. Inspire profunda y lentamente el rocío, mientras oprime el inhalador.
6. Si lo prefiere, puede usar un tubo de extensión entre el inhalador y la boca.
7. Contenga el aire lo más que pueda (casi 10 segundos).
8. Sople (exhale) lentamente.
9. Espere de 30 segundos a 1 minuto entre cada inhalación.

Efectos secundarios (molestias)
El medicamento puede causarle palpitaciones, pulso acelerado, mareo, insomnio o náusea.

Otros inhaladores con corticosteroides
1. La medicina es para prevenir ataques de asma. No lo use en caso de emergencia.
2. Puede provocarle una infección ligera por hongo (algodoncillo) en la boca.
3. Para evitar el hongo, enjuáguese la boca o haga buches con agua y escupa después de usar el inhalador.

Las preguntas fundamentales[2]
1. ¿Para qué es esta medicina?
2. ¿Cómo va a usar esta medicina?
3. ¿Cuáles son los efectos secundarios?
4. Quiero confirmar que no se me olvidó nada. Por favor, dígame cómo va a usar esta medicina.

Questions related to asthma[1]

1. In what season of the year is your asthma worse? In spring, summer, fall, or winter?
2. Please, tell me what makes you feel worse.
3. Do you have allergies to plants, for example? To other things?
4. Do you have cough, phlegm, shortness of breath, wheezing, or chest tightness?

Recommendations

Albuterol inhaler (for asthma)

Take (Make) 1 to 2 puffs every 4 to 6 hours if it is necessary for shortness of breath (or in case of emergency).

Directions

1. Remove the cap.
2. Shake it well.
3. Blow out (exhale) slowly.
4. There are two ways to use your inhaler:
    a. Put the inhaler in your mouth. Close your mouth over the device.
    b. Hold the inhaler 1 to 2 inches (2 to 5 centimeters) away from your open mouth.
5. Inhale the aerosolized medicine (spray) deeply and slowly while pressing the inhaler.
6. If you prefer, you can use a spacer (extension tube) between the inhaler and your mouth.
7. Hold your breath as long as possible (about 10 seconds).
8. Blow out (exhale) slowly.
9. Wait 30 seconds to 1 minute between each inhalation.

Side effects

The medication can cause palpitations, accelerated pulse, dizziness, insomnia, or nausea.

Other inhalers with corticosteroids

1. The medicine is to prevent asthma attacks. Do not use it in case of emergency.
2. It can cause (you) a slight fungal (cotton-like) infection in the mouth.
3. To avoid the fungus, rinse your mouth or swish (make swishes) with water and spit after using the inhaler.

Prime questions[2]

1. What is this medication for?
2. How are you going to use this medication?
3. What are the side effects?
4. I want to make sure I didn't forget anything. Please tell me how you are going to use this medicine.

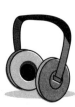

Diálogos para el audio

FARMACÉUTICA: Buenas tardes. Soy la Dra. Clark. ¿Cómo puedo ayudarle?

PACIENTE: *Buenas tardes. Sabe que soy asmática, y se me dificulta respirar en ocasiones. Esta mañana fui a ver al médico. Me revisó y me dio esta receta para un nuevo inhalador. También quiero resurtir mi receta de albuterol.*

FARMACÉUTICA: Por supuesto, señorita.

PACIENTE: *¿Se usa este nuevo inhalador como el de albuterol?*

FARMACÉUTICA: Sí, le voy a dar algunas instrucciones. Pero primero quiero hacerle algunas preguntas.

Preguntas con respecto al asma[1]

1. ¿En qué época del año le empeora el asma? ¿En la primavera, el verano, el otoño o durante el invierno?
   Pues, ahora es otoño y me siento peor con el asma. También en la primavera me siento muy mal.

2. Por favor, dígame con qué se siente peor.
   Bueno, con el pelo de las mascotas, con el polvo y con el cambio de clima.

3. Tiene alergias a las plantas, a los ácaros del polvo, al moho, a la caspa animal o a irritantes como el humo, los limpiadores químicos o aerosoles, por ejemplo? ¿A otras cosas?
   Sí, todas estas cosas me molestan mucho. Ya no tengo en la casa plantas ni animales. El doctor me recomendó que aspirara muy bien mi casa.

4. ¿Tiene tos, flema, falta de aliento, un silbido al respirar u opresión en el pecho?
   Sí, tengo tos y una opresión muy fuerte en el pecho. Me falta mucho la respiración.

Recomendaciones

Pues, estos inhaladores deben ayudarle a sentirse mejor. Primero tiene albuterol que es para la falta de aliento. Haga de 1 a 2 inhalaciones cada 4 a 6 horas, si es necesario, cuando sienta que le falta el aire. El segundo inhalador es un corticosteroide que se llama fluticasona que previene los ataques de asma. Pero tiene que usarlos por algunas semanas para que le dé resultados. Haga 2 inhalaciones dos veces al día.

Instrucciones

Use los dos inhaladores de la misma forma. Le muestro cómo usarlos. Luego, quiero que me muestre cómo los va a usar.
1. Quite la tapa.
2. Agítelo bien.
3. Sople lentamente.
4. Coloque el inhalador de 1 a 2 pulgadas afuera de la boca abierta.
5. Inspire profunda y lentamente el rocío, mientras oprime el inhalador.
6. Si lo prefiere, puede usar un tubo de extensión entre el inhalador y la boca.
7. Contenga el aire lo más que sea posible, si puede, por 10 segundos.
8. Sople lentamente.

9. Espere de 30 segundos a 1 minuto entre cada inhalación.

Efectos secundarios (molestias)

1. El albuterol puede causarle palpitaciones, pulso acelerado, mareo, insomnio o náusea.
2. El corticosteroide le puede provocar una infección ligera por hongo en la boca.

Otras recomendaciones

Para prevenir el hongo, enjuáguese la boca o haga buches con agua y escupa después de usar el corticosteroide. En caso de un ataque de asma, sólo use albuterol.

Las preguntas fundamentales[2]

Para confirmar que le di bien las instrucciones, dígame . . .
1. ¿Para qué son estas medicinas?
   Este inhalador es albuterol para la falta de aliento. Y éste es un corticosteroide para prevenir los ataques.

2. ¿Cómo va a usar los inhaladores?
   Del albuterol, voy a tomar de 1 a 2 inhalaciones cada 4 a 6 horas si es necesario para la falta de aliento. Del otro inhalador, voy a hacer 2 inhalaciones dos veces al día.

   ¿Y cómo los va a usar? Es muy importante usarlos correctamente.
   Ah, primero, agito bien el inhalador. Soplo lentamente. Coloco el inhalador de 1 a 2 pulgadas de la boca abierta. Después, inspiro profunda y lentamente mientras oprimo el inhalador. Contengo el aire lo más que sea posible. Soplo lentamente. Espero de 30 segundos a 1 minuto entre cada inhalación.

3. ¿Cuáles son los efectos secundarios?
   El albuterol me puede causar palpitaciones. El otro inhalador me puede causar un algodoncillo.

4. Quiero confirmar que no se me olvidó nada. Por favor dígame cómo va a usar esta nueva medicina.
   Sí, claro. El nuevo inhalador es para prevenir ataques de asma. Hago 2 inhalaciones dos veces al día. Es buena idea enjuagarme la boca con agua para evitar que se forme una infección de la boca.

Pues excelente. Espero que se sienta mejor con las medicinas.

Gracias, doctora. Le agradezco sus consejos.

Que le vaya bien.

Igualmente.

▇ *Audio dialogues*

PHARMACIST: Good afternoon. I am Dr. Clark. How can I help you?

PATIENT: *Good afternoon. You know that I suffer from asthma, and it's quite difficult for me to breathe on occasions. This morning I went to see the doctor. He checked me and gave me this prescription for a new inhaler. Also, I want to refill my prescription for albuterol.*

PHARMACIST: Yes, of course.

PATIENT: *Do you (Does one) use this new inhaler like the albuterol (one)?*

PHARMACIST: Yes, I am going to give you some directions. But first I want to ask (make) you some questions.

Questions related to asthma[1]

1. At what time of the year does your asthma worsen? In spring, summer, fall, or during the winter?
   Well, now it is fall, and I feel worse with the asthma. Also, in the spring I feel very bad.

2. Please, tell me what makes you feel worse.
   Okay (good), with pet hair, with dust, and with the change in weather.

3. Do you have allergies to plants, to dust mites, to mold, to animal dander, or to irritants like smoke, household cleaners, or aerosols, for example? To other things?
   Yes, all of these things bother me a lot. I no longer have in the house plants or (nor) animals. The doctor recommended (to me) that I vacuum very well my house.

4. Do you have cough, phlegm, shortness of breath, wheezing, or chest tightness?
   Yes, I have cough and a very strong tightness in my chest. I have a lot of shortness of breath.

Recommendations

Well, these inhalers should help you to feel (yourself) better. First, you have the albuterol, which is for shortness of breath. Take (Make) 1 to 2 puffs every 4 to 6 hours if necessary when you feel shortness of breath. The second inhaler is a corticosteroid that is called fluticasone, which prevents asthma attacks. But you have to use them for several weeks to get results. Take (Make) 2 puffs twice a day.

Directions

Use the two inhalers in the same way. I will show you how to use them. Later, I want you to show me how you are going to use them.
1. Remove the cap.
2. Shake it well.
3. Blow out slowly.
4. Place the inhaler 1 to 2 inches away from your open mouth.
5. Inhale the aerosolized medicine (spray) deeply and slowly while pressing the inhaler.
6. If you prefer, you can use a spacer (extension tube) between the inhaler and your mouth.
7. Hold (Contain) your breath as long as possible, if you can, for 10 seconds.
8. Blow out slowly.
9. Wait 30 seconds to 1 minute between each inhalation.

Side effects

1. The albuterol can cause you palpitations, accelerated pulse, dizziness, insomnia, or nausea.
2. The corticosteroid can provoke (in you) a light fungal infection in the mouth.

Other recommendations

To prevent a fungus, rinse your mouth or swish (make swishes) with water, and spit after using the corticosteroid. In case of an asthma attack, use only the albuterol.

Prime questions[2]

To confirm that I gave you good directions, tell me . . .
1. What are these medications for?
   This inhaler is albuterol for shortness of breath. And this is a corticosteroid to prevent the attacks.

2. How are you going to use these inhalers?
   For the albuterol, I am going to take 1 to 2 puffs every 4 to 6 hours if it is necessary for shortness of breath. For the other inhaler, I am going to take (make) 2 puffs two times a day.

   And how will you use them? It is very important that you use them correctly.
   Oh, first, I shake well the inhaler. I blow out slowly. I place the inhaler 1 to 2 inches away from my open mouth. Afterward, I breathe in deeply and slowly while I press the inhaler. I hold (contain) my breath (the air) as long as possible. I blow out slowly. I wait from 30 seconds to 1 minute between each inhalation.

3. What are the side effects?
   The albuterol can cause me palpitations. The other inhaler can cause me a fungal infection.

4. I want to make sure I didn't forget anything. Please tell me how you are going to use this new medicine.
   Yes, of course. The new inhaler is to prevent asthma attacks. I take (make) 2 puffs two times a day. It is a good idea to rinse my mouth with water to keep an infection from forming in the mouth.

Well, excellent. I hope that you feel better with the medicines.

Thank you, Doctor. I appreciate your advice.

May you go well.

Likewise (Equally).

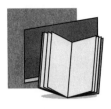

Lección 2   Atomizador nasal
Lesson 2   Nasal spray

Recomendaciones[3]

Atomizador de oximetazolina 0.05% (al cero punto cero cinco por ciento)

Haga de 2 a 3 inhalaciones dos veces al día para la congestión nasal.
1. Sóplese (Suénese) la nariz suavemente.
2. Agite el atomizador suavemente.
3. Póngaselo en la nariz.
4. Cierre la otra fosa nasal oprimiéndola con un dedo.
5. Respire por la nariz.
6. Oprima el atomizador mientras inhala.
7. Repita todos los pasos con la otra fosa nasal.

Efectos secundarios (molestias)

La medicina le puede provocar irritación nasal, insomnio, alta presión o pulso acelerado.

Consejos adicionales

1. No use el atomizador más de 3 a 5 días.
2. Jamás use el atomizador en otra persona.

Etiquetas del producto

1. Para la nariz. (Vía de administración: nasal.)
2. Uso exclusivo del paciente. (Sólo para uso personal.)
3. Agítelo bien.

Las preguntas fundamentales[2]

1. ¿Para qué es esta medicina?
2. ¿Cómo va a usar esta medicina?
3. ¿Cuáles son los efectos secundarios?
4. Quiero confirmar que no se me olvidó nada. Por favor dígame cómo va a usar esta medicina.

Recommendations[3]

Oxymetazoline 0.05% spray

Take 2 to 3 inhalations two times a day for nasal congestion.

1. Gently blow your nose.
2. Shake the spray gently.
3. Insert it (device) into your nose.
4. Close the other nostril, pressing it with a finger.
5. Breathe through the nose.
6. Press the spray while inhaling.
7. Repeat all of the steps with the other nostril.

Side effects

The medication can cause nasal irritation, insomnia, high blood pressure, or increased pulse.

Additional advice

1. Do not use the spray more than 3 to 5 days.
2. Never use the spray on another person.

Product labeling

1. For the nose. (Means of administration: nasal.)
2. For exclusive use of the patient. (Only for personal use.)
3. Shake well.

Prime questions[2]

1. What is this medication for?
2. How are you going to use this medication?
3. What are the side effects?
4. I want to make sure I didn't forget anything. Please tell me how you are going to use this medicine.

Diálogos para el audio

PACIENTE: *Buenas noches. Mi nombre es Lilia Ortiz Quesada. ¿Es usted la farmacéutica?*

FARMACÉUTICA: Sí, efectivamente, Sra. Ortiz. Mi nombre es Verónica Paz y soy la farmacéutica. ¿Cómo la puedo ayudar?

PACIENTE: *Mucho gusto, Dra. Paz. Mire, tengo la nariz pero bien tapada, no puedo ni respirar bien. Estoy muy congestionada. Ya tengo varios días con un resfrío muy fuerte.*

FARMACÉUTICA: Lo siento, Sra. Ortiz. La congestión nasal usualmente la causa un virus y a veces, es por el uso excesivo de ciertos medicamentos. Generalmente desaparece por sí sola en una semana. ¿Está usando algún medicamento?

PACIENTE: *No, no he usado nada, solamente remedios caseros y un analgésico para la calentura. Necesito algo que me alivie la congestión.*

FARMACÉUTICA: Bueno, le puedo recomendar un medicamento que le mejore la congestión.

PACIENTE: *Muchas gracias.*

Recomendaciones[3]

Voy a recomendarle unas gotas de oximetazolina al 0.05%. Haga de 2 a 3 inhalaciones dos veces al día para aliviar la congestión nasal.

1. Suénese la nariz.
2. Agite el atomizador.
3. Póngaselo en la nariz.
4. Cierre la otra fosa nasal oprimiéndola con un dedo.
5. Respire por la nariz.
6. Oprima el atomizador mientras inhala.
7. Repita todos los pasos con la otra fosa nasal.

Consejos adicionales

1. Es muy importante que no use el atomizador más de 3 a 5 días.
2. Jamás use el atomizador de otra persona, ni preste el suyo. Es sólo para uso personal.
3. Tome mucho líquido como té y caldo. Además, un consomé de pollo caliente puede ser de especial ayuda.

Efectos secundarios (molestias)

Esta medicina le puede provocar irritación nasal, insomnio, alta presión o pulso acelerado.

Etiquetas del producto

Es sólo para la nariz.

Las preguntas fundamentales[2]

Bueno, para terminar, me gustaría hacerle algunas preguntas.

1. ¿Para qué es esta medicina?
   Esta medicina es un espray para la nariz tapada.

2. ¿Cómo va a usar esta medicina?
   Voy a hacer de 2 a 3 inhalaciones dos veces al día para la congestión nasal. Primero me sueno la nariz. Después, agito el atomizador. Me lo pongo en la nariz. Me tapo la otra nariz con un dedo. Respiro por la nariz y aprieto el atomizador.

3. Muy bien. ¿Cuáles son las molestias que puede causarle esta medicina?
   La medicina me puede provocar irritación de la nariz o quitarme el sueño.

4. Quiero confirmar que no se me olvidó nada. Por favor dígame cómo va a usar esta medicina.
   Sí, claro. Puedo usarla dos veces al día. Pero no debo de usarla más de 3 a 5 días.

Bueno, que se sienta mejor pronto. Que le vaya bien.

Gracias, Dra. Paz. Es muy amable.

◼ *Audio dialogues*

PATIENT: *Good evening. My name is Lilia Ortiz Quesada. Are you the pharmacist?*

PHARMACIST: Yes, that's correct, Mrs. Ortiz. My name is Verónica Paz, and I am the pharmacist. How can I help you?

PATIENT: *Nice to meet you, Dr. Paz. You see, I have my nose all stopped up, and I can't really breathe well. I am very congested. I have (already) had a cold for several days.*

PHARMACIST: I am sorry, Mrs. Ortiz. A virus usually causes nasal congestion, and sometimes it is because of excessive use of some medications. Generally, it goes away on its own in about a week. Are you using some medication?

PATIENT: *No, I haven't used anything (nothing), only home remedies and an analgesic for the fever. I need something that will alleviate (for me) the congestion.*

PHARMACIST: Good, I can recommend a medication that can improve (for you) the congestion.

PATIENT: *Many thanks.*

Recommendations[3]

I am going to recommend (to you) some oxymetazoline 0.05% drops. Take (Make) 2 to 3 inhalations two times a day to alleviate the nasal congestion.

1. Blow your nose.
2. Shake the spray.
3. Insert it into your nose.
4. Close the other nostril, pressing it with a finger.
5. Breathe through the nose.
6. Press the spray while inhaling.
7. Repeat all of the steps with the other nostril.

Additional advice

1. It is very important that you do not use the spray more than 3 to 5 days.
2. Never use the spray of another person, nor loan yours. (It is) only for personal use.
3. Drink lots of liquid like tea and soup. Moreover, hot chicken broth can be of particular help.

Side effects

This medication can cause you nasal irritation, insomnia, high blood pressure, or rapid pulse.

Product labeling

It is only for the nose.

Prime questions[2]

Good, to end, I would like to ask you (make) some questions.

1. What is this medication for?
   This medicine is a spray for nasal congestion.

2. How are you going to use this medication?
   I am going to take (make) 2 to 3 inhalations two times a day for nasal congestion. First, I blow my nose. Then, I shake the spray. I put it in my nose. I close the other nose with a finger. I breathe through the nose, and I squeeze the spray.

3. Very good. What are the bothersome effects this medicine can cause?
   This medication can cause irritation of the nose or get rid of sleep.

4. I want to make sure I didn't forget anything. Please tell me how you are going to use this medicine.
   Yes, of course. I can use it two times a day. But I should not use it for more than 3 to 5 days.

Good, may you feel better soon. That all goes well.

Thank you, Dr. Paz. You are very kind.

De la cultura / About the culture

1. In Latin America, it is still common to smoke in front of children and pregnant women because there is less awareness of the effects of secondhand smoke.
2. The terms for shortness of breath are "la falta de respiración" or "la falta de aliento." Sometimes patients may also say "la falta de aire," but this expression may also mean to feel suffocated.

Apuntes de gramática / Grammar notes

Impersonal phrases Many phrases that precede a verb express a suggestion or recommendation.
When a general recommendation is made, the infinitive may be used.
When a recommendation is made directly to another person, the subjunctive may be used. The subjunctive mode often includes the word "que."

Infinitive	Es necesario <u>dejar</u> de fumar.	*It is necessary <u>to quit</u> smoking.*
Subjunctive	Es necesario <u>que (usted) deje</u> de fumar.	*It is necessary <u>that you quit</u> smoking.*

Other phrases

Infinitive	Es mejor <u>tomar</u> la medicina.	*It is better <u>to take</u> the medicine.*
Subjunctive	Es mejor <u>que tome</u> la medicina.	*It is better <u>that you take</u> the medicine.*
Infinitive	Es recomendable <u>ir</u> con el doctor.	*It is recommended <u>to go to</u> the doctor.*
Subjunctive	Es recomendable <u>que vaya</u> con el doctor.	*It is recommended <u>that you go</u> to the doctor.*

Ejercicios / Exercises

I. Escriba una pregunta para cada respuesta. (Write a question for each answer.)

1. _____

   Generalmente, mi asma empeora durante la primavera y el otoño.

2. _____

   Puede usar el inhalador de albuterol si siente dificultad para respirar.

3. _____

   Puede causarle algunos efectos secundarios, por ejemplo, palpitaciones y pulso acelerado.

4. _____

   Le recomiendo un atomizador nasal de oximetazolina al 0.05% para la congestión.

5. _____

   Puede provocarle algodoncillo (una infección bucal causada por un hongo).

6. _____

   Puede usar el inhalador de dos maneras: una es introduciéndolo a la boca y la otra es colocándolo a
   1 o 2 pulgadas de la boca.

II. Llene los espacios en blanco con las formas correctas de los verbos. (Fill in the blanks with the correct form of the verbs.)

1. (deber, usar) ¿Cómo _____ _____ el inhalador?

2. (poder, enjuagar[se], usar) ¿_____ _____ la boca después de _____ el inhalador?

3. (sentir, faltar) A veces _____ que me _____ la respiración.

4. (creer, provocar) _____ que el inhalador me está _____ algodoncillo.

5. (agitar, colocar) _____ bien el inhalador y _____ lo de 1 a 2 pulgadas (de 2 a 5 cm)
   de la boca.

6. (oprimir, inhalar, contener) _____ el inhalador mientras _____ y después
   _____ la respiración lo más que sea posible.

III. Escoja la mejor descripción para cada palabra. (Choose the best description for each word.)

1. ____ exhalar   a. no poder respirar por alguna razón

2. ____ sonarse la nariz   b. sentir la nariz tapada

3. ____ algodoncillo   c. sacar el aire de los pulmones al exterior

4. ____ contener la respiración   d. dispositivo para transformar un líquido en un rocío (en gotas muy pequeñas)

5. ____ falta de respiración   e. aparato pequeño

6. ____ atomizador   f. introducir aire en los pulmones

7. ____ palpitaciones   g. limpiarse la nariz por dentro

8. ____ dispositivo   h. sensación muy fuerte de las pulsaciones del corazón, principalmente en las sienes

9. ____ congestión nasal   i. infección por hongos de la boca

10. ____ inhalar   j. dejar de respirar voluntariamente

IV. Conteste las preguntas. (Answer the questions.)

1. ¿Cuáles son algunas cosas que pueden provocar el asma?

2. ¿Cuáles son algunos síntomas del asma?

REFERENCES

1. Bollmeier SG, Prosser TR. Asthma. In: Berardi RR, Kroon LA, McDermott JH, et al., eds. *Handbook of Nonprescription Drugs.* 15th ed. Washington, DC: American Pharmacists Association; 2006:243–61.

2. Gardner M, Boyce RW, Herrier RN. *Pharmacist–Patient Consultation Program PPCP-Unit I: An Interactive Approach to Verifying Patient Understanding.* New York: Pfizer Educational Services; 1991.

3. Scolaro KL. Disorders related to cold and allergy. In: Berardi RR, Kroon LA, McDermott JH, et al., eds. *Handbook of Nonprescription Drugs.* 15th ed. Washington, DC: American Pharmacists Association; 2006:201–28.

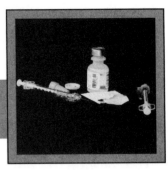

Inyecciones subcutáneas
Subcutaneous injections

Verbos / Verbs		Presente / Present tense			
		Yo	Él, ella, usted	Mandato	Ejemplo
asegurar(se)	to be certain	me aseguro	se asegura	Asegúrese	*Asegúrese de que las unidades estén correctas.*
girar	to roll, to rotate	giro	gira	Gire	*Gire el frasco entre las manos.*
inyectar(se)	to inject	(me) inyecto	se inyecta	Inyéctese	*Inyéctese en el muslo.*
observar	to observe	observo	observa	Observe	*Observe si hay burbujas en la jeringa.*
orinar	to urinate	orino	orina	Orine	*¿Orina mucho?*
pellizcar(se)	to pinch (oneself)	(me) pellizco	(se) pellizca	Pellízquese	*Pellízquese el muslo.*
revisar	to revise, to check	reviso	revisa	Revise	*Revise su nivel de azúcar.*
sacar	to take out	saco	saca	Saque	*Saque el aire de la jeringa.*

Sustantivos / Nouns

la aguja	needle
el aire	air
el azúcar	sugar
el bocadillo	snack
la burbuja	bubble
la cena	dinner, evening meal
el desayuno	breakfast
la extracción	extraction
el frasco ámpula	injectable vial
la galleta salada	salted cracker
la gasa	gauze
el glucómetro	glucometer
la hiperglicemia, la hiperglucemia	hyperglycemia
la hipoglicemia, la hipoglucemia	hypoglycemia
la insulina	insulin
la jeringa	syringe
el jugo	juice
la mezcla	mixture
el nivel	level
el refresco	soft drink
la sed	thirst
la solución	solution (insulin R)
la suspensión	suspension (insulin NPH, 70/30)
la tapa	lid
la tira	strip
la(s) unidad(es)	unit(s)

Adjetivos / Adjectives

alto(a)	high
bajo(a)	short
chico(a)	small
opaco(a)	opaque

Otras expresiones / Other expressions

demasiado(a)	too much, too many
en ayunas	fasting
nunca	never
nunca jamás	never ever
va justo debajo	just go under

Instrucciones / Directions

atrás	back
(a)dentro	inside
a través	across, through
(en)frente	in front
hacia	toward
subcutánea	subcutaneous

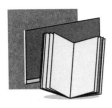

La inyección de insulina
Insulin injection

Preguntas sobre los síntomas de hiperglucemia o hiperglicemia (exceso de azúcar en la sangre)[1]

1. ¿Ha tenido demasiada sed o hambre?
2. ¿Ha tenido la piel reseca?
3. ¿Orina con frecuencia o mucho durante la noche?
4. ¿Se ha revisado el azúcar con un glucómetro?

Recomendaciones

1. Esta insulina es una mezcla de insulina NPH (ene, pe, hache) e insulina R (erre).
2. Se llama insulina 70/30 (setenta sobre treinta). Es para la diabetes.
3. Inyéctese 10 unidades en la mañana 30 minutos antes del desayuno. Por la noche, inyéctese 5 unidades 30 minutos antes de la cena.
4. Esta inyección va justo debajo de la piel (es subcutánea).

Otras presentaciones

1. La insulina en suspensión es opaca.
2. La insulina en solución es clara.

Extracción de la insulina

1. Lávese las manos con agua y jabón.
2. Gire el frasco (ámpula) entre las manos (si se inyecta insulina opaca). Nunca agite el frasco de insulina.
3. Limpie la tapa del frasco con una gasa con alcohol.
4. Jale el émbolo hacia abajo (para llenarlo de aire) hasta _____ unidades.
   La cantidad de aire en la jeringa debe ser igual a la cantidad de insulina que se va a inyectar.
5. Introduzca la aguja dentro del frasco.
6. Empuje el émbolo (para introducir el aire en el frasco).
7. Jale el émbolo suavemente hacia abajo _____ unidades (para sacar la medicina).
8. Asegúrese de que tiene el número correcto de unidades de insulina.
9. Observe si hay burbujas de aire en la jeringa. Si hay burbujas, entonces quítelas (empujándolas con el émbolo).

Inyección de insulina

1. Las áreas para aplicar la inyección son: el estómago, detrás de los brazos (en la parte de arriba) o la parte superior (de arriba) de los muslos.
2. Limpie un área pequeña con una gasa con alcohol.
3. Pellízquese la piel.
4. Introduzca la aguja a través de la piel.
5. Empuje el émbolo hacia adentro (para introducir la medicina).
6. Saque la aguja de la piel.
7. Tire la jeringa en una caja de plástico duro.

Efectos secundarios (molestias):
Hipoglucemia o hipoglicemia (nivel demasiado bajo de azúcar en la sangre)

Esta medicina puede causarle temblor, pulso acelerado, sudor, mareo, dolor de cabeza, cansancio, hambre o debilidad debido al nivel demasiado bajo de azúcar en la sangre.

Otras precauciones

Si siente que tiene un nivel de azúcar muy bajo, usted puede . . .
   . . . tomar un vaso chico de jugo o un refresco regular.
   . . . comer de 2 a 3 galletas saladas o un bocadillo muy chico.
Revise su nivel de azúcar.

Las preguntas fundamentales[2]

1. ¿Para qué es esta medicina?
2. ¿Cómo va a usar esta medicina?
3. ¿Cuáles son los efectos secundarios?
4. Quiero confirmar que no se me olvidó nada. Por favor, dígame cómo va a usar esta medicina.

Questions about the symptoms of hyperglycemia (excess sugar in the blood)[1]

1. Have you had too much thirst or hunger?
2. Have you had dry skin?
3. Do you urinate frequently (with frequency) or a lot during the night?
4. Have you checked your sugar with a glucometer?

Recommendations

1. This insulin is a mixture of insulin NPH and insulin R.
2. It is called insulin 70/30. It is for diabetes.
3. Inject yourself (with) 10 units in the morning 30 minutes before breakfast. At night, inject 5 units 30 minutes before dinner (evening meal).
4. This injection goes just under the skin (it is subcutaneous).

Other formulations

1. Insulin in suspension is opaque.
2. Insulin in solution is clear.

Insulin extraction

1. Wash your hands with water and soap.
2. Roll the (injectable) vial between your hands (if you inject opaque insulin). Never shake the insulin vial.
3. Clean the top of the vial with an alcohol swab (gauze).
4. Pull the plunger down (to fill it with air) to _____ units.
   The amount of air in the syringe should be equal to the amount of insulin that you are going to inject.
5. Insert the needle into the vial.
6. Push the plunger (to put [introduce] air into the vial).
7. Pull the plunger gently down to _____ units (to take out the medicine).
8. Make sure that you have the correct number of units of insulin.
9. Look to see if there are air bubbles in the syringe. If there are bubbles, then get rid of them (by pushing the plunger).

Insulin injection

1. The areas for giving (applying) the injection are the stomach, the back of the arms (in the upper part), or the top of (the front of) the thighs.
2. Clean a small area with an alcohol swab (gauze).
3. Pinch (your) the skin.
4. Insert the needle through the skin.
5. Push the plunger in (to introduce the medicine).
6. Take the needle out of the skin.
7. Throw away the syringe in a hard plastic container.

Side effects:
Hypoglycemia (low blood sugar)

This medication can cause trembling, rapid pulse, sweating, dizziness, headache, fatigue, hunger, or weakness because of a very low level of sugar in the blood.

Other precautions

If you feel that you have a very low blood sugar level, you can . . .
    . . . drink a small glass of juice or a regular soft drink.
    . . . eat from 2 to 3 salted crackers or a very small snack.
Check your blood sugar level.

Prime questions[2]

1. What is this medication for?
2. How are you going to use this medication?
3. What are the side effects?
4. I want to make sure I didn't forget anything. Please tell me how you are going to use this medicine.

Diálogos para el audio

PACIENTE: *Buenas noches, Dra. Bennett. ¿Cómo está usted?*

FARMACÉUTICA: Muy bien, Sra. Núñez. ¿Qué anda haciendo por aquí?

PACIENTE: *¡Sabe que estoy malísima! Me midieron el azúcar y la traigo muy alta. Aunque estoy tomando la pastilla para la diabetes, no me he puesto la insulina. Tengo miedo de empezarla, porque creo que si lo hago me van a cortar las piernas.*

FARMACÉUTICA: Necesita usar la insulina para controlar el azúcar.

PACIENTE: *Ándele pues. Véndame la insulina.*

FARMACÉUTICA: Primero, quiero hacerle algunas preguntas.

Preguntas sobre los síntomas de hiperglucemia[1]

1. ¿Ha tenido demasiada sed o hambre?
   Sí, tengo mucha sed y hambre todo el tiempo.

2. ¿Ha tenido la piel reseca?
   No.

3. ¿Orina con frecuencia o mucho durante la noche?
   Ay sí. Me la paso en el baño toda la noche.

4. ¿Se ha revisado el azúcar con un glucómetro?
   Últimamente, yo no. Pero en la clínica me dijeron que tenía el azúcar sobre 300.

Recomendaciones

1. Sí, es un nivel alto. Su receta es para esta insulina que es una mezcla de insulina NPH (ene, pe, hache) e insulina R (erre). Se llama insulina 70/30. Le voy a dar las instrucciones.

2. Inyéctese 10 unidades en la mañana 30 minutos antes del desayuno. Por la noche, inyéctese 5 unidades 30 minutos antes de la cena.

3. Esta inyección va justo debajo de la piel (es subcutánea).

Extracción de la insulina

Para preparar la insulina:
1. Lávese las manos con agua y jabón.
2. Gire el frasco ámpula entre las manos. Nunca agite el frasco de insulina.
3. Limpie la tapa del frasco con una gasa con alcohol.
4. Jale el émbolo de la jeringa hacia abajo para llenar la jeringa de aire. La cantidad de aire en la jeringa debe ser igual a la cantidad de insulina que se va a inyectar.
5. Introduzca la aguja dentro del frasco.
6. Empuje el émbolo hacia arriba para introducir el aire en el frasco.
7. Jale el émbolo suavemente hacia abajo para sacar 10 unidades de insulina en las mañanas. En las noches saque 5 unidades.
8. Asegúrese de que tiene el número correcto de unidades de insulina.
9. Observe si hay burbujas de aire en la jeringa. Si hay, entonces quítelas (empujándolas con el émbolo).

No me voy a acordar de tantas cosas.

No se preocupe. Todo va a estar escrito. Le voy a dar las instrucciones para aplicar la inyección.

Inyección de insulina

1. Las áreas para aplicar la inyección son el estómago, detrás de los brazos en la parte de arriba o la parte de arriba de los muslos.
2. Limpie un área pequeña con una gasa con alcohol.
3. Pellízquese la piel.
4. Introduzca la aguja a través de la piel.
5. Empuje el émbolo hacia adentro para introducir la insulina.
6. Saque la aguja de la piel.
7. Tire la jeringa en una caja de plástico duro.

Efectos secundarios (molestias)

La insulina puede tener algunos efectos secundarios. Por ejemplo, puede causarle hipoglicemia que es un nivel demasiado bajo de azúcar en la sangre. Los síntomas son temblores, pulso acelerado, sudor, mareo, dolor de cabeza, cansancio, hambre o debilidad.

¡Ya ve! Me voy a sentir peor.

Claro que no. Pero tiene que seguir bien las instrucciones. Yo le voy a decir cómo mejorar los efectos secundarios.

Otras precauciones

Si siente que tiene un nivel de azúcar muy bajo, usted puede tomar un vaso chico de jugo o refresco regular o comer de 2 a 3 galletas saladas o un bocadillo muy chico. Revise su nivel de azúcar.

Me parece que todo es muy complicado.

Bueno, entonces, para confirmar qué le he dicho, explíqueme . . .

Las preguntas fundamentales[2]

1. ¿Para qué es esta medicina?
   Para la diabetes.

2. ¿Cómo va a usar esta medicina? Muéstreme con la jeringa y la insulina.
   Me voy a inyectar en las mañanas 10 unidades y 5 unidades en las noches, así.

   Muy bien hecho. Pero recuerde que se la debe de poner 30 minutos antes del desayuno y la cena.

3. A ver, dígame ¿Cuáles son los efectos secundarios?
   Pues, me puede dar temblores, hambre, sudor, pulso acelerado o mareo si se me baja mucho el azúcar.

4. Quiero confirmar que no se me olvidó nada. Por favor, dígame otra vez cómo va a usar esta medicina.
   Me voy a inyectar en las mañanas 10 unidades media hora antes de desayunar y 5 unidades en las noches media hora antes de cenar.

Perfecto, Sra. Nuñez. Ya está lista para aplicarse la insulina. Si la usa correctamente, no le va a pasar nada en las piernas. Pero recuerde seguir la dieta y hacer el ejercicio que le recomendó el doctor. También, tiene que tomarse sus pastillas. Llámeme si tiene alguna duda de cómo usar la insulina.

Muchas gracias, doctora. Voy a seguir todas las recomendaciones. Buenas noches.

Que le vaya bien.

Audio dialogues

PATIENT: *Good evening, Dr. Bennett. How are you?*

PHARMACIST: Very good, Mrs. Nuñez. What are you doing here?

PATIENT: *You know, I am really sick! They measured my sugar, and it was very high. Even though I am taking a pill for diabetes, I have not given myself insulin. I am afraid (have fear) to start it because if I do it I believe that they are going to cut off my legs.*

PHARMACIST: You need to use the insulin to control your sugar.

PATIENT: *All right, then. Sell me the insulin.*

PHARMACIST: First, I want to ask you some questions.

Questions about the symptoms of hyperglycemia[1]

1. Have you had a lot of thirst or hunger?
   Yes, I am very thirsty and hungry all of the time.

2. Have you had dry skin?
   No.

3. Do you urinate with frequency or a lot during the night?
   Oh, yes. I go to the bathroom all night.

4. Have you checked your sugar with a glucometer?
   Lately, I have not. But in the clinic, they told me that (I had) my sugar was over 300.

Recommendations

1. Yes, it is a high level. Your prescription is for this insulin that is a mixture of insulin NPH and insulin R. It is called insulin 70/30. I am going to give you instructions.
2. Inject (yourself with) 10 units in the morning 30 minutes before breakfast and 5 units at night 30 minutes before dinner (evening meal).
3. This injection goes just under the skin (it is subcutaneous).

Insulin extraction

To prepare the insulin:
1. Wash your hands with water and soap.
2. Roll the injectable vial between your hands. Never shake the insulin vial.
3. Clean the top of the vial with an alcohol swab (gauze).
4. Pull the plunger down to fill the syringe with air. The amount of air in the syringe should be equal to the amount of insulin that you are going to inject.
5. Insert the needle into the vial.
6. Push the plunger up to insert air into the vial.
7. Pull the plunger gently down to take 10 units of insulin in the mornings. In the evenings, take 5 units.
8. Make sure that you have the correct number of units of insulin.
9. Look to see if there are air bubbles in the syringe. If there are, then get rid of them (by pushing the plunger).

I am not going to remember (myself) so many things.

Don't worry (yourself). Everything is going to be written. I am going to give you the directions to apply the injection.

Insulin injection

1. The areas for giving (applying) the injection are the stomach, in back of the upper part of the arms, or the top of the thighs.
2. Clean a small area with an alcohol swab (gauze).
3. Pinch (your) the skin.
4. Insert the needle through the skin.

5. Push the plunger in to introduce the insulin.
6. Take the needle out of the skin.
7. Throw away the syringe in a hard plastic container.

Side effects

Insulin can have some side effects. For example, it can cause you to have hypoglycemia, which is a very low level of sugar in the blood. The symptoms are trembling, rapid pulse, sweating, dizziness, headache, fatigue, hunger, or weakness.

Look already! I am going to feel (myself) worse.

Of course not. But you have to follow the directions well. I am going to tell you how to improve the side effects.

Other precautions

If you feel that you have a very low blood sugar level, you can drink a small glass of juice or a regular soft drink or eat from 2 to 3 salted crackers or a very small snack. Check your blood sugar level.

It seems to me that everything is very complicated.

Okay, then, to confirm what I have told you, explain to me . . .

Prime questions[2]

1. What is this medication for?
   For diabetes.

2. How are you going to use this medication? Show me with the syringe and the insulin.
   I am going to inject myself in the mornings 10 units, and 5 units in the evenings, like this.

   Very well done. But remember that you should take it (put it in) 30 minutes before breakfast and dinner (evening meal).

3. Let's see, tell me, what are the side effects?
   Well, it can give me trembling, hunger, sweating, rapid pulse, or dizziness if my blood sugar drops a lot.

4. I want to make sure I didn't forget anything. Please tell me again how you are going to use this medicine.
   I am going to inject myself in the mornings 10 units half an hour before eating breakfast and 5 units in the evenings half an hour before eating dinner.

Perfect, Mrs. Núñez. You are ready to apply the insulin (to yourself). If you use it correctly, nothing will happen to your legs. But remember to follow the diet and to exercise as the doctor recommended to you. Also, you have to take your pills. Call me if you have some doubt about how to use the insulin.

Thank you very much, Doctor. I am going to follow all of your recommendations. Good evening.

May you go well.

De la cultura / About the culture

1. Hispanics in the United States are more likely (1.7 times) to have type 2 diabetes than are whites. Many Hispanics are often not aware that they have diabetes.[3]

2. Some patients from the Hispanic community express fear of receiving insulin injections. This fear may arise because patients have family members who experienced amputation or blindness shortly after starting insulin injections. Patients may link injections to amputation or blindness rather than to better control of blood sugar.

3. In Mexico, some regions use the verb "checar" or "chequear" in place of "observar" or "revisar," meaning to observe or check. Patients may say "Tengo que checarme (or chequearme) el azúcar" when they want to express "I have to check my sugar." In some Spanish-speaking circles, "chequear" is considered slang.

4. When providing information about insulin use in Spanish, pharmacists should be aware of the subtleties of time in relationship to meals. For example, the term "almorzar" can mean "to eat breakfast" or "to eat lunch." The term "comer" can be "to eat" or "to eat lunch." Also, in some Hispanic cultures, meals occur at mid-afternoon (about 2:00 or 3:00 p.m.) and later in the evening (about 8:00 or 9:00 p.m.). These different concepts of terms and times open the door for confusion and side effects when injecting insulin. The most precise counseling may need to include the exact time of the day to eat (e.g., 7:00 a.m. and 6:00 p.m.) and provide the relationship to an exact meal (in accordance with the patient's understanding of times to eat during the day).

Ejercicios / Exercises

I. Escriba una pregunta para cada respuesta. (Write a questions for each answer.)

1. ¿_____?
   Siempre use el número correcto de unidades de insulina que indica su receta.

2. ¿_____?
   Sólo gire el frasco de insulina entre las manos; nunca lo agite.

3. ¿_____?
   Introduzca al frasco una cantidad de aire igual al número de unidades que va a sacar y después saque esa cantidad de insulina.

4. ¿_____?
   Observe si hay burbujas de aire en la jeringa y sáquelas empujando el émbolo hacia arriba.

5. ¿_____?
   Las áreas para aplicar la inyección son el estómago, atrás de los brazos y la parte de arriba de los muslos.

6. ¿_____?
   Si tiene síntomas de hipoglucemia (falta de azúcar), tome medio vaso de jugo de naranja o coma una galleta salada.

II. Llene los espacios en blanco con los verbos adecuados. (Fill in the blanks with the appropriate verbs.)

1. (haber, sentir) Tengo mucho malestar. Desde ayer me _____ _____ mareado y muy débil.

2. (estar, aplicar) Me _____ _____ 6 unidades de insulina diariamente.

3. (dar hambre, sentir[se], ir) A veces me _____ muy mal, me ____ _____ y me _____ mareado y _____ al baño con mucha frecuencia.

4. (saber, tener que, sacar, observar) _____ que _____ _____ _____ las unidades correctas de insulina y _____ que no tenga burbujas de aire la jeringa.

5. (necesitar, obtener, jalar) _____ _____ las unidades de insulina _____ el émbolo.

6. (tirar, usar) _____ la jeringa que _____ en una caja de plástico duro.

III. Escoja la mejor descripción para cada palabra. (Select the best description for each word.)

1. _____ aguja   a. oprimir un área de la piel con los dedos

2. _____ émbolo   b. pequeño recipiente de vidrio que contiene la medicina

3. _____ pellizcar   c. parte de la jeringa que se introduce en la piel

4. _____ frasco   d. dispositivo para cubrir los frascos

5. _____ tapa   e. arte de la jeringa que sirve para empujar la medicina

6. _____ unidad   f. dar vueltas a algo

7. _____ girar   g. medida del medicamento

IV. Escriba otras recomendaciones para prevenir problemas con la diabetes (por ejemplo, los pies, la aspirina, las vacunas). (Write other recommendations to prevent problems with diabetes, such as feet, aspirin, vaccinations.)

1. _____

2. _____

3. _____

4. _____

REFERENCES

1. Assemi M, Morello CM. Diabetes mellitus. In: Berardi RR, Kroon LA, McDermott JH, et al., eds. *Handbook of Nonprescription Drugs.* 15th ed. Washington, DC: American Pharmacists Association; 2006:955–94.

2. Gardner M, Boyce RW, Herrier RN. *Pharmacist–Patient Consultation Program PPCP-Unit I: An Interactive Approach to Verifying Patient Understanding.* New York: Pfizer Educational Services; 1991.

3. National Alliance for Hispanic Health. *Delivering Health Care to Hispanics: A Manual for Providers.* 4th ed. Washington, DC: Estrella Press; 2007:124.

El examen físico

Physical exam

Signos vitales / Vital signs[1]

Verbos / Verbs		Presente / Present tense		
		Yo	Él, ella, usted	Mandato
acostar(se)	to lie down (oneself)	me acuesto	se acuesta	Acuéstese
checar	to check	checo	checa	Cheque
descansar	to rest	descanso	descansa	Descanse
enrollar	to roll up	enrollo	enrolla	Enrolle
esperar	to wait, to hope	espero	espera	Espere
guardar silencio	to be quiet	guardo silencio	guarda silencio	Guarde silencio
levantar(se)	to stand (oneself up)	me levanto	se levanta	Levántese
medir	to measure	mido	mide	Mida
morder	to bite	muerdo	muerde	No muerda
observar	to watch, to observe	observo	observa	Observe
pesar	to weigh	peso	pesa	Pese
relajar(se)	to relax oneself	me relajo	se relaja	Relájese
recomendar	to recommend	recomiendo	recomienda	Recomiende
remangar(se)	to roll up sleeves	me remango	se remanga	Remánguese
sentar(se)	to sit (oneself)	me siento	se sienta	Siéntese
sentir(se)	to feel (oneself)	me siento	se siente	—

Sustantivos / Nouns

el apretón	tight squeeze	el peso	weight
el baumanómetro	Sphygmomanometer, blood pressure manometer	el (los) pie(s)	foot (feet)
		la presión arterial	blood pressure
el brazalete del baumanómetro	blood pressure cuff	la pulgada	inch
el corazón	heart	el pulso	pulse
la estatura	height	la(s) respiración(es)	breath, respiration
el estetoscopio	stethoscope	la temperatura	temperature
la libra	pound	el termómetro	thermometer
la medida	measurement		
el oído	ear		
la onza	ounce		

Adjetivos / Adjectives

irregular	irregular
lento(a)	slow
normal	normal
rápido(a)	rapid, fast
regular	regular

Otras expresiones / Other expressions

alrededor del brazo	around the arm
el aparatito	small device
debajo de la lengua	under the tongue
exceso de peso, sobrepeso	overweight
bajo de peso	underweight

Pesos y medidas / Weight and height

1. Voy a pesarlo(la). Pesa _____ libras y _____ onzas.
   I am going to weigh you. You weigh(s) _____ pounds and _____ ounces.

2. Voy a medirlo(la). Mide _____ pies y _____ pulgadas.
   I am going to measure you. You measure _____ feet and _____ inches.

La temperatura / Temperature

1. Voy a tomarle la temperatura.
   I am going to take your temperature.

2. Oral / Oral
   a. Saque la lengua.
      Stick out your tongue.
   b. Voy a ponerle el termómetro debajo de la lengua.
      I am going to put the thermometer under your tongue.
   c. No lo muerda.
      Don't bite it.

3. Por el oído / By ear
   Voy a ponerle este aparatito en su oído.
   I'm going to put this device in your ear.

4. Su temperatura es de _____ grados fahrenheit.
   Your temperature is _____ degrees Fahrenheit.

5. Es normal.
It is normal.
Tiene algo de calentura.
You have somewhat of a fever.
Tiene fiebre (o mucha calentura).
You have a fever (or a high fever).

Preguntas / Questions

1. ¿Ha fumado en los últimos 30 minutos?
Have you smoked in the past 30 minutes?

2. ¿Ha tomado bebidas con cafeína durante los últimos 30 minutos? (ejemplos: ¿refrescos, té o café?)
Have you had any caffeinated drinks in the past 30 minutes (examples: soft drinks, tea, or coffee)?

3. ¿Está tomando algún medicamento?
Are you taking any medication?

El pulso / Pulse

1. Voy a tomarle el pulso.
I'm going to check (take) your pulse.

2. Relájese por favor.
Relax, please.

3. Espere un momentito.
Wait a few seconds.

4. Su pulso es de _____ (pulsaciones por minuto).
Your pulse is _____ (beats every minute).

5. Es bueno.
It is good.
Es un poco rápido.
It is a little fast.
Es un poco lento.
It is a little slow.

Las respiraciones / Respiration

1. Estoy observando sus respiraciones.
I am watching your breathing.

2. Tiene casi ____ respiraciones por minuto.
You breathe about ____ breaths per minute.

3. Su respiración es regular.
Your breathing is regular.
Está respirando un poco rápido.
You are breathing a little fast.

La presión arterial / Blood pressure

1. Voy a tomarle (checarle) la presión.
I'm going to take (check) your blood pressure.

2. Siéntese.
Sit down.
Levántese.
Stand up.
Acuéstese.
Lie down.

3. Por favor, ponga los dos pies en el piso.
   Please put both feet on the floor.

4. Relájese. Descanse un momento.
   Relax. Rest a moment.

5. Por favor guarde silencio.
   Please be quiet.

6. Enróllese la manga. (Remánguese.)
   Roll up your sleeve.

7. Va a sentir un apretón en el brazo.
   You will feel a tight squeeze on your arm.

8. Su presión arterial es de 120/80 (ciento veinte sobre ochenta).
   Your blood pressure is 120/80 (120 over 80).

Ejercicios / Exercises

1. **Practique en voz alta las siguientes medidas y después deletréelas.** (Practice saying the following measurements aloud and then spell them.)

Pesos:	*Ejemplo: 12 lbs 4 oz*	doce libras y cuatro onzas
8 lbs 14 oz		_____
59 lbs		_____
106 lbs		_____
191 lbs		_____
221 lbs		_____

Medidas:	*Ejemplo: 4′ 11″*	cuatro pies y once pulgadas
23″		_____
3′ 8″		_____
5′ 10″		_____

Temperatura:	*Ejemplo: 99°*	noventa y nueve grados
98.6°		_____
100°		_____
102°		_____
37°		_____
40°		_____

Pulso:	*Ejemplo: 64*	sesenta y cuatro pulsaciones por minuto
60		_____
75		_____
83		_____
92		_____

Respiraciones:	*Ejemplo: 14*	catorce respiraciones por minuto
12		_____
16		_____
18		_____
20		_____

Presión arterial:	*Ejemplo: 143/88*	ciento cuarenta y tres sobre (por) ochenta y ocho
115/68		_____
120/80		_____
136/94		_____
158/102		_____

2. **¿Qué le puede recomendar a un paciente que tiene una presión de 150/92?** (What can you recommend to a patient who has a blood pressure of 150/92?)

3. **¿Qué le puede recomendar a un paciente que tiene una presión de 182/98?** (What can you recommend to a patient who has a pressure of 182/98?)

4. **¿Qué cambios en el estilo de vida le puede recomendar al paciente para mejorar su presión?** (What lifestyle changes can you recommend to a patient to improve his or her blood pressure?)

El oído, la nariz y la garganta / Ear, nose, and throat[2]

Verbos / Verbs		Presente / Present tense		
		Yo	Él, ella, usted	Mandato
abrir	to open	abro	abre	Abra
doler	to hurt	me duele(n)	le duele(n)	—
escuchar	to listen	escucho	escucha	Escuche
hablar	to talk	hablo	habla	Hable
oír	to hear	oigo	oye	Oiga
palpar	to palpate	palpo	palpa	Palpe
perder	to lose	pierdo	pierde	Pierda
seguir	to continue	sigo	sigue	Siga
revisar	to check	reviso	revisa	Revise
tocar	to touch	toco	toca	Toque

Otras palabras / Other words

las anginas, las amígdalas	tonsils	el oído	ear
la boca	mouth	la oreja	outer ear
la campanilla, la úvula	uvula	el (la) otorrinolaringólogo(a)	ear, nose, and throat doctor
el cerumen, la cerilla	earwax	el otoscopio	otoscope
el cuello	neck	el pómulo	cheekbone
el ganglio, el nódulo linfático	lymph node	los senos nasales	nasal sinuses
la garganta	throat	el tímpano	tympanic membrane
la nariz	nose	la tiroides	thyroid

Problemas de salud / Health problems

el catarro	runny nose
la congestión nasal	nasal congestion
el fuego en la boca	mouth sores
la hinchazón	swelling
la infección del oído	ear infection
la mudez	muteness
la pérdida del oído	hearing loss
el resfrío	cold
la rigidez	stiffness
la sinusitis	sinusitis
la sordera	deafness

El examen / Exam

Voy a checarle los oídos, la nariz y la garganta.
I'm going to check your ears, nose, and throat.

Los oídos / Ears

1. ¿Ha perdido el oído? ¿Puede oír o escuchar bien?
   Have you had any loss of hearing? Can you hear or listen well?

2. ¿Ha tenido dolor de oídos?
   Have you had earaches?

3. Voy a revisarle los oídos.
   I am going to check your ears.

La nariz y los senos nasales / Nose and sinuses

1. ¿Ha tenido congestión nasal?
   Have you felt congested?

2. Voy a tocarle este lado de la nariz. Siga respirando.
   I'm going to touch this side of your nose. Continue breathing.

3. Ahora del otro lado.
   Now the other side.

4. Voy a tocarle la cara. ¿Tiene hinchazón en esta área? ¿En estas áreas? ¿Le duele?
   I'm going to touch your face. Do you have swelling in this area? In these areas? Does it hurt (you)?

5. Voy a ponerle una luz en los pómulos.
   I'm going to put this light on your cheekbones.

La boca / Mouth

1. ¿Ha tenido fuegos en la boca?
   Have you had any mouth sores?

2. ¿Ha tenido dolor de garganta?
   Have you had a sore throat?

3. ¿Tiene dificultad para hablar?
   Do you have difficulty speaking?

3. Abra la boca.
   Open your mouth.

4. Diga "Ah."
   Say "Ah."

El cuello / Neck

1. ¿Ha sentido rigidez en el cuello?
   Have you felt stiffness in your neck?

2. Voy a checarle el cuello.
   I'm going to check your neck.

3. Voy a revisarle la tiroides.
   I'm going to check your thyroid.

Ejercicio / Exercise

Dé una recomendación a los padres de un bebé para prevenir las infecciones de los oídos.
(Give a recommendation to the parents of a baby to prevent ear infections.)

El examen de los pulmones / Lung exam[3]

Verbos / Verbs		Presente / Present tense		
		Yo	Él, ella, usted	Mandato
contener	to contain	contengo	contiene	Contenga
exhalar	to breathe out	exhalo	exhala	Exhale
inhalar	to inhale	inhalo	inhala	Inhale
inspirar	to inspire	inspiro	inspira	Inspire
levantar(se)	to stand up (oneself)	me levanto	se levanta	Levántese
respirar	to breathe	respiro	respira	Respire
sacar	to take out	saco	saca	Saque
soplar	to blow	soplo	sopla	Sople

Sustantivos / Nouns

el aliento	breath, air in lungs	el medidor de flujo máximo pulmonar	peak flow meter
la auscultación	auscultation		
la costilla	rib	el pulmón (los pulmones)	lung(s)
el esternón	sternum, breast bone	la pulsación	pulsation
el medidor de aliento	peak flow meter	la zona (verde, amarilla, roja)	zone (green, yellow, red)

Adjetivos / Adjectives

cianótico(a)   cyanotic

Problemas de salud del aparato respiratorio / Respiratory system health problems

el asma	asthma	la EPOC (enfermedad pulmonar obstructiva crónica)	COPD (chronic obstructive pulmonary disease)	la infección respiratoria	respiratory infection
la bronquitis	bronchitis			la pulmonía	pneumonia
la cianosis	cyanosis			el resfrío	cold
el enfisema pulmonar	emphysema	la gripe	influenza	la tos	cough
				la tuberculosis	tuberculosis

El Examen / Exam

Voy a revisar y escuchar sus pulmones.
I am going to check and listen to your lungs.

1. Inhale profundamente y contenga la respiración.
   Inhale deeply and hold your breath.

2. Respire normalmente.
   Breathe normally.

3. Exhale completamente. Saque todo el aire.
   Breathe out as fully as possible. (Take out all of the air.)

El medidor de aliento / Peak flow meter

1. Levántese.
   Stand up.

2. Ponga el indicador en la base de la escala.
   Slide the marker to the bottom of the scale.

3. Inhale tan profundo como le sea posible. Inhale profundamente.
   Inhale as fully as possible. Inhale deeply.

4. Sople fuerte. Exhale tan rápido y completamente como pueda.
   Blow out hard. Exhale as fast and fully as you can.

5. Repita este proceso dos veces más.
   Repeat this process two more times.

6. Escriba el valor más alto.
   Write down the highest value.

Ejercicio / Exercise

Explíquele a un asmático cuáles deben ser sus metas de volumen respiratorio (zonas verde, amarilla y roja).
(Explain to an asthmatic what should be his or her respiratory volume goals [green, yellow, and red zones].)

El examen del corazón / Heart exam[4]

Verbos / Verbs — Presente / Present tense

		Yo	Él, ella, usted	Mandato
morir	to die	muero	muere	—
latir	to beat	—	late, me late	—

Sustantivos / Nouns

el (la) cardiólogo(a)	cardiologist	el ECG de esfuerzo (o prueba de esfuerzo)	stress test	el marcapasos	pacemaker
el cateterismo cardíaco	cardiac catheterization			el pulso	pulse
la cirugía de derivación coronaria	bypass surgery	la ecocardiografía	echocardiogram	el estent coronario	stent
		el electrocardiograma	electrocardiogram, EKG		

Problemas de salud del sistema cardiovascular / Cardiovascular system health problems

la angina de pecho	angina	el colesterol alto	high cholesterol	la presión alta	high blood pressure
la angioplastía	angioplasty	el derrame cerebral, la embolia, la hemorragia cerebral	stroke	el puente coronario	coronary bypass
la apoplejía	stroke				
las arterias obstruidas	clogged arteries			el soplo	murmur
el ataque cardíaco, el ataque al corazón	heart attack	la hipertensión	hypertension	el trasplante de corazón	heart transplant
la aterosclerosis	atherosclerosis	la insuficiencia cardíaca congestiva	congestive heart failure		
el coágulo	clot				

Las partes del sistema cardiovascular / Parts of the cardiovascular system

la arteria	artery	la válvula	valve	pulmonar	pulmonary (lungs)
la aurícula	atrium	tricúspide	tricuspid (right)		
la vena	vein	bicúspide o mitral	bicuspid or mitral (left)	aórtica	aortic (body)
el ventrículo	ventricle				

El examen / Exam

Voy a revisar y escuchar su corazón.
I am going to check and listen to your heart.

1. Por favor acuéstese.
   Please lie down.

2. Por favor siéntese.
   Please sit down.

3. Guarde silencio por favor.
   Please be quiet.

Ejercicios / Exercises

1. **Explíquele a un paciente qué condiciones de salud pueden provocarle un ataque al corazón.** (Explain to a patient what health conditions can cause a heart attack.)

2. **Escriba algunos síntomas de un ataque al corazón.** (Write some of the symptoms of a heart attack.)

3. **Escriba algunos síntomas de una embolia.** (Write some of the syptoms of a stroke.)

El examen de los pies para pacientes diabéticos / Diabetic foot exam[5]

Verbos / Verbs		Presente / Present tense		
		Yo	Él, ella, usted	Mandato
arder(se)	to burn oneself	me arde(n)	le arde(n)	—
cerrar	to close	cierro	cierra	Cierre
checar(se)	to check oneself	me checo	se checa	Chéquese
dormir(se un pie)	to fall asleep (foot)	se me duerme (el pie)	se le duerme	—
explicar	to explain	le explico	le explica	Explíqueme
hormiguear	to tingle (like ants)	me hormiguea(n)	le hormiguea(n)	—
picar(se)	to pinch	me pico, me pica	se pica, le pica	Píquese
quitar(se)	to take off	me quito	se quita	Quítese
revisar(se)	to check oneself	me reviso	se revisa	Revísese

Sustantivos / Nouns

el dedo del pie	toe	el tobillo	ankle
el pie	foot	la uña	nail
la planta del pie	sole	el vello	body hair (foot)
el pulso	pulse		

Adjetivos / Adjectives

agudo(a)	sharp	sordo(a)	dull
caliente	hot, warm	seco(a)	dry
frío(a)	cold	tibio(a)	lukewarm
limpio(a)	clean		

Problemas de salud de los pies diabéticos / Diabetic foot health problems

la ampolla	blister	la falta de sensibilidad	lack of sensation	la neuropatía	neuropathy
la amputación	amputation	en los pies	in the feet	la picazón	intense itching
la circulación	circulation	la herida	wound	el piquete	stick, bite
la comezón	itching	la infección	infection	la úlcera	ulcer
el dolor (de pies)	foot pain	la llaga	sore	la uña enterrada	ingrown nail

El examen / Exam

1. ¿Tiene dolor o ardor en sus piernas?
   Do you have pain or burning in your legs?

2. ¿Tiene los pies fríos muy seguido?
   Are your feet cold very often?

3. ¿Tiene alguna cortada, herida, llaga o úlcera en los pies? ¿Desde cuándo?
   Do you have a cut, wound, sore, or ulcer on your feet? Since when?

4. ¿Le pican, le hormiguean o se le duermen los pies?
   Do your feet pinch you, tingle (like ants), or feel like they fall asleep?

5. Voy a revisarle (checarle) los pies.
   I am going to check your feet.

6. Por favor, quítese los zapatos y los calcetines (las medias).
   Please take off your shoes and socks (hose).

7. Cierre los ojos. ¡No haga trampa!
   Close your eyes. Don't cheat!

8. Cuando sienta un piquetito, diga sí.
   When you feel a "little stick," say yes.

9. Dígame si puede sentir esto.
   Tell me if you can feel this.

10. Voy a revisarle (checarle) la circulación y los pulsos de los pies.
    I am going to check the circulation and the pulses in your feet.

11. Sus pies se ven sanos.
    Your feet look good (healthy).

    Tal vez, tenga algunos problemas en los pies. Vaya con el doctor pronto.
    You may have a few problems with your feet. Go to your doctor soon.

12. Revísese los pies cada día (diariamente, a diario, todos los días).
    Check your feet every day.

Complicaciones / Complications

1. Puede tener neuropatías (problemas de la sensibilidad de los nervios o falta de sensación) en sus pies.
   You may have neuropathics (nerve sensitivity problems or loss of sensation) in your feet.

2. Puede tener mala circulación en los pies.
   You may have bad circulation in your feet.

3. Puede necesitar una amputación.
   You may need an amputation.

Ejercicio / Exercise

Explíquele a un diabético cómo cuidarse los pies. (Explain to a diabetic how to take care of his or her feet.)

Inmunizaciones y vacunas / Immunizations and vaccinations[6]

Verbos / Verbs		Presente / Present tense		
		Yo	Él, ella, usted	Mandato
enrollar(se)	to roll up	me enrollo	se enrolla	Enróllese
inyectar(se)	to inject (oneself)	me inyecto	se inyecta	Inyéctese
relajar(se)	to relax	me relajo	se relaja	Relájese

Las enfermedades / Illnesses

la bacteria, de bacteria	bacteria	la neumonía	pneumonia	las vacunas muertas	killed vaccines
la difteria	diphtheria	las paperas, la parotiditis	mumps	las vacunas vivas	live vaccines
la gripe	influenza	la poliomielitis, la polio	polio	la varicela, la viruela loca	chicken pox
la hepatitis	hepatitis	el refuerzo búster (popular)	booster		
la influenza	influenza	la rubéola	rubella	viral (de virus)	viral
la influenzae haemophilus tipo B	Haemophilus influenzae type B	el sarampión	measles	la viruela	smallpox
		el tétanos	tetanus	el virus del papiloma humano (VPH)	human papilloma virus (HPV)
		la tosferina	pertussis		
el meningocócico	meningococcus	la vacuna, la inmunización	immunization		

Los signos y síntomas del choque anafiláctico / Signs and symptoms of anaphylactic shock

la comezón	itchiness
la dificultad para respirar	difficulty breathing
las ronchas	hives
el salpullido	rash

Preguntas e instrucciones / Questions and directions

1. ¿Está enfermo(a) hoy?
   Are you sick today?

2. ¿Tiene alguna alergia a algo? ¿Es alérgico(a) a los huevos? ¿A los cacahuates (al maní)?
   Do you have allergies to anything? Are you (male/female) allergic to eggs? To peanuts?

3. ¿Está embarazada?
   Are you pregnant?

4. ¿Ha tenido problemas (reacción alérgica) con alguna vacuna?
   Have you had problems (allergic reaction) with some vaccines?

5. Siéntese.
   Sit down.

6. Por favor enróllese la manga.
   Please roll up your sleeve.

7. Relaje el brazo.
   Relax your arm.

8. Lo (la) voy a inyectar. Va a sentir un piquete.
   I am going to inject you. You will feel a stick.

9. Espere aquí 15 a 20 minutos, por favor.
   Wait here for 15 to 20 minutes, please.

Ejercicio / Exercise

Revise el sitio del Internet de CDC o http://www.immunize.org. Busque información en español sobre las vacunas. Escriba cuáles son algunos de los efectos secundarios relacionados con las vacunas. (Review the CDC Internet site or http://www.immunize.org. Look for information in Spanish on vaccines. Write down some of the frequent side effects related to vaccines.)

REFERENCES

1. Seidel HM, Ball JW, Dains JE, et al., eds. *Mosby's Guide to Physical Examination.* 4th ed. St. Louis: Mosby, Inc; 1999:55–60.
2. Seidel HM, Ball JW, Dains JE, et al., eds. *Mosby's Guide to Physical Examination.* 4th ed. St. Louis: Mosby, Inc; 1999:308–51.
3. Seidel HM, Ball JW, Dains JE, et al., eds. *Mosby's Guide to Physical Examination.* 4th ed. St. Louis: Mosby, Inc; 1999:352–408.
4. Seidel HM, Ball JW, Dains JE, et al., eds. *Mosby's Guide to Physical Examination.* 4th ed. St. Louis: Mosby, Inc; 1999:409–85.
5. Seidel HM, Ball JW, Dains JE, et al., eds. *Mosby's Guide to Physical Examination.* 4th ed. St. Louis: Mosby, Inc; 1999:76–7, 409–85.
6. Immunization Action Coalition. Screening questionnaire for adult immunization. Available at: http://www.immunize.org/catg.d/p4065.pdf. Accessed June 1, 2008.

Tiempo
Time

La división del tiempo / Divisions of time

el segundo	second
el minuto	minute
la hora	hour
el día	day
la semana	week
el mes	month
la estación	season
el año	year
el año bisiesto	leap year

Los días de la semana / Days of the week

el lunes / los lunes	Monday / every Monday
el martes / los martes	Tuesday / every Tuesday
el miércoles / los miércoles	Wednesday / every Wednesday
el jueves / los jueves	Thursday / every Thursday
el viernes / los viernes	Friday / every Friday
el sábado / los sábados	Saturday / every Saturday
el domingo / los domingos	Sunday / every Sunday
el fin de semana / los fines de semana	weekend(s)

Los meses del año / Months of the year

enero	January	julio	July
febrero	February	agosto	August
marzo	March	septiembre	September
abril	April	octubre	October
mayo	May	noviembre	November
junio	June	diciembre	December

Las estaciones del año / Seasons of the year

el invierno	winter	el verano	summer
la primavera	spring	el otoño	fall

Los colores / Colors

amarillo(a)	yellow	morado(a)	purple
anaranjado(a)	orange	negro(a)	black
azul	blue	rojo(a)	red
blanco(a)	white	rosa	pink
café	brown	verde	green

Examples*

camis**as** duraz**no** (peach-colored shirts [plural feminine])	NOT	camis**as** durazn**as**
vestid**os** naranj**a** (orange fruit-colored dresses [plural masculine])	NOT	vestid**os** naranj**os**
corbat**as** vin**o** (wine-colored ties [plural feminine])	NOT	corbat**as** vin**as**

Examples

pastill**as** anaranjad**as** (orange-colored pills [plural feminine])
car**ro** anaranjad**o** (orange-colored car [singular masculine])
botell**as** azul**es** (blue-colored bottles [plural no gender])

Descripciones / Descriptions

chico(a)	little		oscuro(a)	dark
claro(a)	clear		pálido(a)	pale
duro(a)	thick (or hard material)		pequeño(a)	little
espeso(a)	thick		redondo(a)	circular
flojo(a)	thin (or lazy)		con sangre	with blood
grande	big		seco(a)	dry
líquido(a)	runny		sólido(a)	thick, solid
manchado(a)	spotted		transparente	clear, transparent
mojado(a)	wet		viscoso(a)	thick, viscous

Los números / Numbers

0 cero	1 uno†	2 dos	3 tres	4 cuatro
5 cinco	6 seis	7 siete	8 ocho	9 nueve
10 diez	11 once	12 doce	13 trece	14 catorce
15 quince	16 dieciséis	17 diecisiete	18 dieciocho	19 diecinueve
20 veinte	21 veintiuno†	22 veintidós	23 veintitrés	24 veinticuatro
25 veinticinco	26 veintiséis	27 veintisiete	28 veintiocho	29 veintinueve
30 treinta	31 treinta y uno†	32 treinta y dos	33 treinta y tres	34 treinta y cuatro
35 treinta y cinco	36 treinta y seis	37 treinta y siete	38 treinta y ocho	39 treinta y nueve

---

*In Spanish, colors derived from the name of objects (e.g., fruit, beverages) do not take a plural form and do not add or change a feminine "a" or masculine "o" at the end of the word. For example, one might describe an item as the color of a strawberry (**fresa**), an avocado (**aguacate**), or red wine (**vino**). If more than one item is involved (plural), an "s" or "es" would not be added in the Spanish language. Neither would the feminine or masculine endings be added.

†"Uno" is shortened to "un" before masculine singular nouns.

Examples:	Un medicamento	One medication
	Veintiún frascos	Twenty-one vials
	Treinta y un estudiantes	Thirty-one students

10 diez	**100** cien	**1,000** mil*	**1,000,000** un millón
20 veinte	**200** doscientos	**2,000** dos mil	
30 treinta	**300** trescientos	**3,000** tres mil . . .	
40 cuarenta	**400** cuatrocientos		
50 cincuenta	**500** quinientos		
60 sesenta	**600** seiscientos	**80,000** ochenta mil	
70 setenta	**700** setecientos	**200,000** doscientos mil	
80 ochenta	**800** ochocientos	**600,000** seiscientos mil	
90 noventa	**900** novecientos		

101 ciento uno
102 ciento dos
201 doscientos uno

Los números ordinales / Ordinal numbers

primero(a)†	first	sexto(a)	sixth
segundo(a)	second	séptimo(a)	seventh
tercero(a)	third	octavo(a)	eighth
cuarto(a)	fourth	noveno(a)	ninth
quinto(a)	fifth	décimo(a)	tenth

¿Qué hora(s) es (son)? / What time is it?

Es (Son) la(s) ___	It is _____	y media	30 minutes
A las _____	At _____	y cuarto	15 minutes
Es la hora	It is time	cuarto para	15 minutes to
minuto(s)	minute(s)	Falta(n) ___ para las ___	It is ___ to ___

de la mañana	in the morning	a las 8 de la mañana	at 8 in the morning
de la tarde	in the afternoon		
de la noche	at night		

por la mañana	during the morning	mañana por la mañana	tomorrow during the morning
por la tarde	during the afternoon		
por la noche	during the night		

Examples

Es la una y media.	It is 1:30.
Son las once y cuarto (11:15) de la mañana.	It is 11:15 in the morning.
A las 7:40.	At 7:40.
Al cuarto para las ocho.	At a quarter to eight.
Falta un cuarto para las seis.	It is a quarter to six.
Faltan quince minutos para las nueve.	It is fifteen minutes until nine.
Son las nueve menos quince.	It is nine minus fifteen minutes (8:45).

In many parts of Latin America, military time is used, particularly for social events in the afternoon or evening.

Example	Son las trece horas.	It is 13:00 / 1 p.m.

---

*To indicate "thousands," the Spanish language uses a period (e.g., 1.000), whereas the English language uses a comma (e.g., 1,000). If a decimal point is needed in Spanish, then a comma is used for a decimal (e.g., 1.000,50). This form is opposite to the English usage. For the purposes of this text, the authors will avoid using this format to prevent confusion and medical errors in dosing. However, a patient who is writing a number may use a period or comma in a different manner.

†The forms "primer" and "tercer" are used before masculine singular nouns only.

Example:	el primer tratamiento	the first treatment
	el primer pasillo	the first aisle
	el tercer piso	the third floor

Expresiones interrogativas / Interrogative expressions

¿Cómo?	How?	¿Dónde?	Where?
¿Cómo se dice . . . ?	How does one say . . . ?	¿Adónde?	To where?
¿Cuál?	What? Which?	¿De dónde?	From where?
¿Cuál es?	Which one is?	¿Para qué?	For what?
¿Cuáles son?	Which ones are?	¿Por qué?	Why?
¿Cuándo?	When?	¿Por qué no?	Why not?
¿Desde cuándo?	Since when?	¿Qué?	What?
¿A qué hora?	At what time?	¿Quién(es)?	Who? Whom?
¿Cuánto(a)? ¿Cuántos(as)?	How many? How often?		

Preguntas para clarificar / Questions for clarification

¿Mande?*	What? (Please repeat.)
¿Cómo dice? ¿Cómo dijo?	What did you say? What?
¿Dígame? Dígame otra vez.	What? (Tell me.) Tell me again.
¿Perdón?	Excuse me? (Please repeat.)

Note: Some phrases may be used differently in various parts of Latin America.

---

*When something is not understood, it may be considered impolite in Spanish to say "¿Qué?" for *What?* It is more appropriate to say "¿Mande?" or "Dígame otra vez."

Gramática
Grammar

Verbos / Verbs

The following section provides grammar notes on the more commonly used verb tenses studied in the text, with clear emphasis in the pharmacy setting. This section is not designed to be a comprehensive review of grammar but rather provides insight on how verbs are conjugated and placed within sentence constructions that are useful in everyday speech.

The grammar is divided into the following sections:
1. Conjugation of **ser** and **estar** (present, past, and imperfect tenses)
2. Verbs in the present tense
3. Commands
4. Future progressive (**ir** + a + infinitive)
5. Compound verbs
6. Present perfect tense (**haber** + past participle)
7. Present progressive tense (**estar** + present progressive)

Ser / To be (existence—permanent conditions)

	Singular			Plural		
Present	Yo	**soy**	I am	Nosotros(as)	**somos**	We are
	Tú	**eres**	You are (familiar)			
	Él, Ella, Usted	**es**	He is, She is, You are (formal)	Ellos, Ellas, Ustedes	**son**	They are, You are
Past	Yo	**fui**	I was	Nosotros(as)	**fuimos**	We were
	Tú	**fuiste**	You were (familiar)			
	Él, Ella, Usted	**fue**	He was, She was, You were (formal)	Ellos, Ellas, Ustedes	**fueron**	They were, You were
Imperfect	Yo	**era**	I used to be	Nosotros(as)	**éramos**	We used to be
	Tú	**eras**	You used to be (familiar)			
	Él, Ella, Usted	**era**	He used to be, She used to be, You used to be (formal)	Ellos, Ellas, Ustedes	**eran**	They used to be, You used to be

Estar / To be (location, feeling—temporary conditions)

		Singular			**Plural**	
Present	Yo	**estoy**	*I am*	*Nosotros(as)*	**estamos**	*We are*
Present	Tú	**estás**	*You are (familiar)*			
Present	Él, Ella, Usted	**está**	*He is, She is, You are (formal)*	*Ellos, Ellas, Ustedes*	**están**	*They are, You are*
Past	Yo	**estuve**	*I was*	*Nosotros(as)*	**estuvimos**	*We were*
Past	Tú	**estuviste**	*You were (familiar)*			
Past	Él, Ella, Usted	**estuvo**	*He was, She was, You were (formal)*	*Ellos, Ellas, Ustedes*	**estuvieron**	*They were, You were*
Imperfect	Yo	**estaba**	*I used to be*	*Nosotros(as)*	**estábamos**	*We used to be*
Imperfect	Tú	**estabas**	*You used to be (familiar)*			
Imperfect	Él, Ella, Usted	**estaba**	*He used to be, She used to be, You used to be (formal)*	*Ellos, Ellas, Ustedes*	**estaban**	*They used to be, You used to be*

Verbos en tiempo presente / Verbs in the present tense

In Spanish, all the verbs in the infinitive form have a stem and a different ending: -ar, -er, -ir. Most Spanish verbs are regular, and the conjugations in their different tenses follow the general rules. However, some verbs are irregular in some of their tenses. Below is an example of the present tense conjugation of some regular and irregular verbs.

Examples of verbs

Infinitive	Stem	Ending
hablar (*to talk*)	habl-	-ar
beber (*to drink*)	beb-	-er
vivir (*to live*)	viv-	-ir

Regular verbs

The stem does not change when conjugating the verb in present tense. The endings change depending on the subject (e.g., I, you, the medicine) and the type of ending (-ar, -er, or -ir).

Summary of endings for present tense

Ending			Singular		Plural	
-ar	hablar					
		Yo	habl **o**	*Nosotros(as)*	habl **amos**	
		Tú	habl **as**			
		Él, Ella, Usted	habl **a**	*Ellos, Ellas, Ustedes*	habl **an**	
-er	beber					
		Yo	beb **o**	*Nosotros(as)*	beb **emos**	
		Tú	beb **es**			
		Él, Ella, Usted	beb **e**	*Ellos, Ellas, Ustedes*	beb **en**	
-ir	vivir					
		Yo	viv **o**	*Nosotros(as)*	viv **imos**	
		Tú	viv **es**			
		Él, Ella, Usted	viv **e**	*Ellos, Ellas, Ustedes*	viv **en**	

Present tense regular verbs ending in -ar   Example: **hablar** (to talk)

		Stem	Ending	
Singular	*Yo*	**habl-**	**-o**	*I talk*
	Tú	**habl-**	**-as**	*You (familiar) talk*
	Él, Ella, Usted	**habl-**	**-a**	*He talks, She talks, You (formal) talk*
Plural	*Nosotros(as)*	**habl-**	**-amos**	*We talk*
	Ellos, Ellas, Ustedes	**habl-**	**-an**	*They talk, You (all) talk*

Present tense regular verbs ending in -er   Example: **beber** (to drink)

		Stem	Ending	
Singular	*Yo*	**beb-**	**-o**	*I drink*
	Tú	**beb-**	**-es**	*You (familiar) drink*
	Él, Ella, Usted	**beb-**	**-e**	*He, drinks, She drinks, You (formal) drink*
Plural	*Nosotros(as)*	**beb-**	**-emos**	*We drink*
	Ellos, Ellas, Ustedes	**beb-**	**-en**	*They drink, You (all) drink*

Present tense regular verbs ending in -ir   Example: **vivir** (to live)

		Stem	Ending	
Singular	*Yo*	**viv-**	**-o**	*I live*
	Tú	**viv-**	**-es**	*You (familiar) live*
	Él, Ella, Usted	**viv-**	**-e**	*He lives, She lives, You (formal) live*
Plural	*Nosotros(as)*	**viv-**	**-imos**	*We live*
	Ellos, Ellas, Ustedes	**viv-**	**-en**	*They live, You (all) live*

Present tense irregular verbs

The stem may change when conjugating the verb in present tense. Each type of irregular verb has particular rules. We highly recommend looking for the correct stem changes of any new verb in a dictionary of verbs, especially when in doubt.

Irregular verbs   Example: **decir** (to say)

		Stem	Ending	
Singular	*Yo*	**dig-**	**-o**	*I say*
	Tú	**dic-**	**-es**	*You (familiar) say*
	Él, Ella, Usted	**dic-**	**-e**	*He says, She says, You (formal) say*
Plural	*Nosotros(as)*	**dec-**	**-imos**	*We say*
	Ellos, Ellas, Ustedes	**dic-**	**-en**	*They say, You (all) say*

Los mandatos / Commands

The command form of verbs is highly useful in the pharmacy setting because it is an effective and respectful way to give directions to patients.

For example: <u>*Tome*</u> *la medicina todos los días.*   <u>*Take*</u> *your medicine every day.*
                 <u>*Dígame*</u> *dónde le duele.*   <u>*Tell me*</u> *where you hurt.*

Pharmacists are usually talking with adult patients or other health care professionals. Therefore, when conveying instructions, it is proper to address a patient or professional formally as *Usted* or a group of persons as *Ustedes*.

Regular verb endings for the command form are the following:
    -ar verbs change to the ending "-e" or "-en"
    -er and -ir verbs change to the ending "-a" or "-an"

The stem may change in the command form as found in the present tense for the first person singular *Yo* (I).

Regular verb endings in the command form

	Usted	Ustedes
-ar	-e	-en
-er	-a	-an
-ir	-a	-an

Examples of regular verbs in the command form for the formal "you"

	Verb	Usted You (formal singular)	Ustedes You (formal plural)
-ar	**tomar** (to take, to drink)	Tom<u>e</u> la medicina cada 4 horas. *Take the medicine every 4 hours.*	No la tom<u>en</u> con comida. *Don't take it (the medicine) with food.*
	regresar (to return)	Regres<u>e</u> el próximo martes. *Return next Tuesday.*	No regres<u>en</u> mañana. *Don't return tomorrow.*
-er	**beber** (to drink)	Beb<u>a</u> mucha agua. *Drink a lot of water.*	No beb<u>an</u> alcohol. *Don't drink alcohol.*
	comer (to eat)	No com<u>a</u> durante la mañana. *Don't eat during the morning.*	Com<u>an</u> después de tomar la medicina. *Eat after you take the medicine.*
-ir	**abrir** (to open)	Abr<u>a</u> la botella, *Open the bottle.*	No abr<u>an</u> el supositorio. *Don't open the suppository.*
	decir (to say, tell)	Dig<u>a</u> las instrucciones. *Say the directions.*	¡No me dig<u>an</u>! *Don't tell me (You all must be joking).*

Futuro progresivo / Future progressive

Future progressive   (ir + "a" + infinitivo)   <u>**Voy a tomar**</u> la medicina.
                      (to be going + infinitive)   <u>*I am going to take*</u> *the medicine.*

The future progressive is a common and useful way to conjugate verbs for the future tense. Pharmacy personnel will find this verb tense to be a convenient way to communicate with the patient when in need of information about the future.

For example, a pharmacist or technician might ask:
    ¿Va a regresar más tarde?   *Are you going to return later?*

The patient may say:
    Voy a seguir las instrucciones.   *I am going to follow the directions.*

The future progressive is made up of the present tense conjugation of the verb "**ir**" plus the preposition "**a**" followed by the infinitive of the main verb to be used in the future tense. In English, the equivalent of this type of conjugation is expressed as "*to be going to . . .*"
    Ir (*to be going*) + a + *infinitive*

Present tense of **ir** (*to go*)

Pronoun	Present tense
Yo	**voy**
Tú	**vas**
Él, Ella, Usted	**va**
Nosotros(as)	**vamos**
Ellos, Ellas, Ustedes	**van**

Examples:

Voy + a + comer	*I am going*	+	*to eat (infinitive verb)*
Va + a + ver	*You are going*	+	*to see (infinitive verb)*

Verbos compuestos / Compound verbs

When two verbs are used together in a sentence, a compound verb or auxiliary (helping) verb is often used. The first verb "helps" the second verb. Only the first verb is conjugated; the second verb remains in the infinitive (original) form.

For example: necesitar (to need) + comprar (to buy) = necesito comprar (I need to buy)

Compound verb		Yo	Usted
deber	to have to (must)	Debo beber . . . *I must drink . . .*	Debe ser . . . *You must be . . .*
necesitar	to need	Necesito tomar . . . *I need to take . . .*	Necesita asistir . . . *You need to attend . . .*
poder	to be able to (can)	Puedo comer . . . *I can eat . . .*	Puede ver . . . *You can see . . .*
querer	to want	Quiero saber . . . *I want to know . . .*	Quiere ir . . . *You want to go . . .*
tener (que)	to have (to)	Tengo que esperar . . . *I have to wait . . .*	Tiene que regresar . . . *You have to return . . .*

Examples:

1. Debo beber ocho vasos de agua al día.
   I must drink eight glasses of water daily.
2. Puede ver al doctor la próxima semana.
   You can see the doctor next week.
3. Necesito tomar mi medicina a las 3 de la tarde.
   I need to take my medicine at 3 in the afternoon.
4. El paciente quiere venir a consulta mañana mismo.
   The patient wants to come for a consultation in the morning.
5. Tiene que regresar el martes a recoger su medicina.
   You have to return Tuesday to pick up your medicine.

Presente perfecto / Present perfect

Present perfect	(haber + past participle)	<u>He tenido</u> fiebre desde ayer.
	(to have + past participle)	*<u>I have had</u> a fever since yesterday.*

The use of the present perfect tense is helpful in the pharmacy setting because it can describe how a patient has been feeling or what the patient has been doing about a condition. The time frame of the present perfect is understood as the immediate past up to the present moment.

For example, patients may say:

<u>He tenido</u> tos desde hace 3 días.	*<u>I have had</u> a cough since 3 days ago.*
<u>He estado</u> enfermo por 10 días.	*<u>I have been</u> sick for 10 days.*

The pharmacist might ask:

¿<u>Ha visto</u> al doctor?	*Have you seen the doctor?*
¿<u>Ha tomado</u> alguna medicina?	*Have you taken any medicine?*

The present perfect tense in Spanish is the exact equivalent to the present perfect in English. It uses the conjugated forms of the verb "haber" (*to have*) plus the past participle of the main verb. The verb "to have," in this case, is only an auxiliary (helping) verb.

In Spanish, to form the present perfect, first conjugate the verb "haber" in its present tense. These conjugated forms of the verb "haber" should agree with the subject.

Haber

Pronoun	Present tense
Yo	he
Tú	has
Él, Ella, Usted	ha
Nosotros(as)	hemos
Ellos, Ellas, Ustedes	han

Then, to create the past participle, change the ending (-ar, -er, -ir). All the regular verbs ending in **-ar** have the past participle ending **-ado**. For those regular verbs ending in -er or -ir, the past participle ending is **-ido**.

Past participle conjugation for regular verbs

	-ar	-er	-ir
Past participle	-ado	-ido	-ido

Regular verbs in the past participle

Together, the present tense conjugation of "haber" with the regular verb in the past participle takes the following form:

Person	Present tense "haber"	Past participle -ar	Past participle -er	Past participle -ir
Yo	he *I have*	habl **ado** *spoken*	ten **ido** *had*	ven **ido** *come*
Tú	has *You (familiar) have*	trabaj **ado** *worked*	com **ido** *eaten*	viv **ido** *lived*
Él, Ella, Usted	ha *He has, She has, You (formal) have*	cur **ado** *cured*	escog **ido** *chosen*	surt **ido** *filled*
Nosotros(as)	hemos *We have*	est **ado** *been*	s **ido** *been*	sufr **ido** *suffered*
Ellos, Ellas, Ustedes	han *They have, You have*	evit **ado** *avoided*	pod **ido** *been able to*	ido *gone*

Some verbs are irregular in the past participle. The following are some verbs whose endings are irregular in the past participle.

Irregular verbs in the past participle

Verbos	Verbs	Participio pasado	Past participle
abrir	to open	abierto	opened
cubrir	to cover	cubierto	covered
decir	to say	dicho	said
devolver	to return	devuelto	returned
escribir	to write	escrito	written
freír	to fry	frito	fried
hacer	to do, to make	hecho	done, made
morir	to die	muerto	died
poner	to put	puesto	put
resolver	to solve	resuelto	solved
romper	to break	roto	broken
satisfacer	to satisfy	satisfecho	satisfied
ver	to see	visto	seen
volver	to come back	vuelto	come back

Presente progresivo / Present progressive

Present progressive	(estar + "gerundio")	Mi hijo <u>está llorando.</u>
	(to be + present participle)	*My son <u>is crying.</u>*

The present progressive tense can be useful to describe what the patient is doing or how the patient is feeling at that very moment. It may also describe how the patient is currently resolving a health problem or issue.

For example, patients may say:
<u>Me estoy sintiendo</u> muy mal. — *<u>I am feeling</u> very bad.*
<u>Le estoy poniendo</u> la crema a mi hija. — *<u>I am putting</u> a cream on my daughter.*

The pharmacist might ask:
¿Qué <u>está tomando</u> para el resfrío? — *What <u>are you taking</u> for your cold?*
¿<u>Está comiendo</u> bien? — *<u>Are you eating</u> well?*

The present progressive tense is the equivalent to the present progressive in English. It uses the conjugated forms of the verb "estar" (*to be* [*temporary state*]) plus the "-ing" form of the main verb (present participle). The verb "to be" in this case is an auxiliary (helping) verb.

In Spanish, to form the present progressive, first conjugate the verb "estar" in its present tense to agree with the subject.

Estar

Pronoun	Present tense
Yo	Estoy
Tú	Estás
Él, Ella, Usted	Está
Nosotros(as)	Estamos
Ellos, Ellas, Ustedes	Están

To make the "-ing" form ("gerundio" in Spanish, or "present participle" in English), change the -ar ending to "-ando" and the -er and -ir endings to "-iendo." Many of the verb endings are regular in this tense, but sometimes the stem of the verb in the present progressive form does change.

Present participle conjugation for regular verbs

	-ar	-er	-ir
"Gerundio" / Present participle ("-ing")	-ando	-iendo	-iendo

Examples of regular verb endings in the present progressive

The conjugated verbs in the present progressive take on the following form.

Person	Present tense "estar"	-ar	-er	-ir
Yo	estoy *I am*	habl **ando** *talking*	ten **iendo** *having*	vin **iendo** *coming*
Tú	estás *You (familiar) are*	trabaj **ando** *working*	com **iendo** *eating*	viv **iendo** *living*
Él, Ella, Usted	está *He is, She is, You (formal) are*	cur **ando** *curing*	escog **iendo** *choosing*	surt **iendo** *filling*
Nosotros(as)	estamos *We are*	s **iendo** *being*	s **iendo** *being*	sufr **iendo** *suffering*
Ellos, Ellas, Ustedes	están *They are, You are*	evit **ando** *avoiding*	pon **iendo** *putting*	sigu **iendo** *following*

Examples of irregular verb endings in the present progressive

A few verbs have **irregular** verb endings in the present progressive.

Verbos	Verbs	Gerundio	Present participle
leer	to read	le yendo	reading
creer	to believe	cre yendo	believing

Glosario español–inglés
Spanish–English glossary

a fondo	thoroughly	aguado(a)	watery
a través	across, through	agudo(a)	sharp
a veces	sometimes	la aguja	needle
abajo	down, below	ahora	now
el abdomen	abdomen	ahora mismo	right now
el aborto natural	miscarriage	ahorita	in a few moments
el aborto provocado	abortion (induced)	el aire	air
		el ajo	garlic
el abrigo	coat	al revés	backward, opposite side
abril	April		
abrir(se)	to open	alcohólico(a)	alcoholic
los ácaros del polvo	dust mites	el alergeno	allergen
las acedías	acidity	la alergia	allergy
el aceite	oil	alérgico(a)	allergic
la acidez	acidity, heartburn	el algodón	cotton
ácido(a)	acid	el algodoncillo (slang)	oral thrush (cotton-like)
el acné	acne		
acostar(se)	to lie down, to go to bed	el aliento	breath, air in lungs
actualmente	currently	la alimentación	usual diet
adentro	inside	la alimentación por sonda	enteral feeding
la adicción	addiction		
adolorido(a)	sore	aliviar(se)	to feel better, to alleviate
el adulto (la adulta)	adult		
la advertencia	warning	alrededor	around
el aerosol	spray (nasal, topical)	alto(a)	high
		el aluminio	aluminum
afectado(a)	affected	amargo(a)	bitter
afectar(se)	to affect	amarillento(a)	yellowish
afuera	outside	amarillo(a)	yellow
agachar(se)	to bend over	las amígdalas	tonsils
agitar	to shake	la ampolla	blister
agosto	August	la ampolleta	ampule
el agrandamiento	enlargement	la amputación	amputation
agrio(a)	sour, acid, tart	el analgésico	analgesic
las agruras	acidity	anaranjado(a)	orange
el agua tibia	lukewarm water	el anestésico	anesthetic

la angina de pecho	angina
las anginas	tonsils
la angioplastía	angioplasty
el año	year
el año bisiesto	leap year
la ansiedad	anxiety
el antebrazo	forearm
los anteojos	eyeglasses
antes (de)	before
el antiácido	antacid
el antibacteriano	antibacterial
el antihistamínico	antihistamine
el antiséptico	antiseptic
aórtico(a)	aortic
el aparatito	small device
el aparato	apparatus, device
el apetito	appetite
el aplicador	applicator
aplicar(se)	to apply, to instill
la apoplejía	stroke
el apoyo	help, support
apretado(a)	tight-fitting
apretar	to squeeze, to press
el apretón	tight squeeze
el arco del pie	arch of the foot
arder(se)	to burn
el área	area
arriba	above
la arteria	artery
las arterias obstruídas	clogged arteries
la articulación	joint
el artículo	item
el ascensor	elevator
el asco	nausea
asegurar(se)	to be certain
las asentaderas	buttocks

el asma	asthma	brillante	bright
aspirar	to vacuum	el bronceador	suntan lotion
el ataque al corazón	heart attack	los bronquios	bronchi
el ataque cardíaco	heart attack	la bronquitis	bronchitis
el ataque de asma	asthma attack	la bufanda	scarf
la aterosclerosis	atherosclerosis	la burbuja	bubble
el atomizador	spray	búster (popular)	booster
atrás	back, behind	el cabello	hair
el aura	aura	la cabeza	head
la aurícula	atrium	la cachucha	cap (baseball)
la auscultación	auscultation	cada	each, every
la avena	oatmeal	la cadera	hip
la axila	axillary	caducar	to expire
ayudar	to help	la caducidad	expiration
el azúcar	sugar	café / el café	brown / coffee
azul	blue	la cafeína	caffeine
la bacteria	bacteria	la caja	cash register/box
bajar	to go down, to lower, to lose (weight)	la caja registradora	cashier's desk
		el cajón	drawer
bajar de peso	to lose (weight)	el calambre	cramp
bajo	under	las calcetas	knee-highs
bajo(a)	short	el(los) calcetín(es)	sock(s)
el baño	bathroom, bath	el calcio	calcium
barato(a)	inexpensive	el caldo	clear broth
la barbilla	chin	calentar	to heat, to warm
el barril	barrel (of inhaler)	la calentura	fever
el barro	blackhead	caliente	hot
la basura	trash	el callo	corn, callus
el baumanómetro	sphygmomano-meter, blood pressure manometer	calmar(se)	to relieve
		cambiar(se)	to change
		el cambio	change (coins)
		caminar	to walk
el bebedero	water fountain	la campanilla	bell, uvula
beber	to drink	el cansancio	fatigue
la bebida	drink	la cantidad	quantity
el bicarbonato de sodio	sodium bicar-bonate	la capa	layer
		la cápsula	capsule
bicúspide o mitral	bicuspid or mitral	la cara	face
el bienestar	comfort, well-being	el(la) cardiólogo(a)	cardiologist
		cargar	to charge
blanco(a)	white	caro(a)	expensive
blancuzco(a)	whitish	el casco	helmet
blando(a)	soft	el caso	case (situation)
el bloqueador de sol	sunblock	la caspa	dandruff
la boca	mouth	la caspa animal	animal dander
boca abajo	lying with your face down	el catarro	runny nose
		cateterismo cardíaco	cardiac catheter-ization
boca arriba	on your back or face up	la causa	cause
		causar	to cause
el bocadillo	snack	la cebolla	onion
los bochornos	hot flashes	la ceguera	blindness
la bolsa	bag	la ceja	eyebrow
la borrachera (slang)	drunkenness	la cena	dinner, evening meal
borracho(a) (slang)	drunk		
borroso(a)	blurry	los centavos	cents
la botella	bottle	el centímetro	centimeter
el brazalete del baumanómetro	blood pressure cuff	el cepillo	brush
		el cerebro	brain
el brazo	arm	la cerilla	earwax

cerrado(a)	closed
cerrar	to close
el cerumen	earwax
el cervix	cervix
el cesto de la basura	trashcan
el champú	shampoo
checar(se)	to check
el cheque	check
el chicle	gum (chewing)
chico(a)	small, little
chupar	to suck on
la cianosis	cyanosis
cianótico(a)	cyanotic
el ciclo	cycle
ciego(a)	blind
la cintura	waist
la circulación	circulation
la cirugía de derivación coronaria	coronary bypass surgery
claro(a)	clear
el coágulo	clot
el codo	elbow
la cola	line
el colesterol alto	high cholesterol
el cólico	abdominal cramp
colocar	to place
el color	color
comenzar	to begin, to start
comer	to eat
la comezón	itching
la comida	food, meal
el comprimido	pill
la computadora	computer
común	common
con	with
con sangre	with blood
condimentado(a)	spicy, seasoned
conectar	to attach
confiable	safe, reliable
confirmar	to confirm
la confusión	confusion
confuso(a)	confused
la congestión del pecho	chest congestion
la congestión nasal	nasal congestion
la conjuntivitis	conjunctivitis
la consistencia	consistency
consultar	to consult
contagiar(se)	to contaminate, to get infected
contener	to contain
contener la respiración	hold the breath
continuo(a)	continuous
contraer	to contract, to acquire a disease
controlar	to control
el corazón	heart
correcto(a)	correct
la cortada	cut
la cortadura	cut

la cosa	thing
la costilla	rib
creer	to believe
la crema	cream, lotion
el crisantemo	chrysanthemum
la cruda (slang)	hangover
el cuarto	room
el cuarto de galón	quart (quarter of a gallon)
cubrir(se)	to cover
la cuchara	tablespoon
la cucharada	tablespoonful
la cucharadita	teaspoonful
la cucharita	teaspoon
el cuello	neck
el cuero cabelludo	scalp
el cuerpo	the body
el cupón	coupon
curar(se)	to cure
el curita	bandage
dañino(a)	damaging, harmful
dar	to give
de costumbre	usually
de tal manera	in such a way
de vez en cuando	sometimes, once in a while
debajo	underneath, below
deber (de)	should, must
la debilidad	weakness
decir	to say, to tell
el dedal de hule	finger cot (rubber)
el (los) dedo(s) de la mano	finger(s)
el (los) dedo(s) del pie	toe(s)
dejar	to permit, to allow, to leave
dejar (de)	to stop, to quit
dejar de fumar	to quit smoking
delgado(a)	thin
demasiado(a)	a lot of, too much
depositar	to deposit
la depresión	depression
deprimido(a)	depressed
deprimir(se)	to get depressed
el (la) derecho(a)	straight, straight ahead, right (direction)
la dermatitis	dermatitis
el derrame cerebral	stroke
el desayuno	breakfast
descansar	to rest
describir	to describe
desde ayer	since yesterday
desechable	disposable
el desecho	discharge
desgrasado(a)	without fat
desinfectar	to disinfect
el desodorante	deodorant
despellejar	to peel (skin)
despertar(se)	to wake up
después (de)	after, later
el desvanecimiento	fainting
el día	day
diariamente	every day, daily
la diarrea	diarrhea
diciembre	December
el diente	tooth
diferente	different
la dificultad	difficulty
la difteria	diphtheria
el dinero	money
directamente	directly
disculpar	to excuse, to be sorry
la disfunción eréctil	erectile dysfunction
disolver	to dissolve
el dispositivo	device
la distensión abdominal	abdominal distension
doler(se)	to hurt / to be in pain
el dolor	pain
el domingo	Sunday
dormir(se)	to sleep
el dorso de la mano	back of the hand
la dosis (las dosis)	dose(s)
la ducha femenina	feminine douche
durante	during
duro(a)	hard, thick
la ebriedad	drunkenness
la ecocardiografía	echocardiogram
la edad	age
el efectivo	cash
efectivo(a)	effective
efervescente	effervescent
el ejercicio	exercise
el electrocardiograma	electrocardiogram, EKG
el elevador	elevator
el elíxir	elixir
el embarazo	pregnancy
la embolia	stroke
el émbolo	plunger (applicator part)
la emergencia	Emergency
emotivo(a)	emotional
el empeine del pie	top of the foot
empeorar	to worsen
empezar	to begin
empujar	to push
la emulsión	emulsion
en ocasiones	at times
las encías	gums
endurecer	to harden
el enema	enema
enero	January
la enfermedad crónica	chronic illness
el enfisema pulmonar	emphysema
enfrente	in front
el engrosamiento	overgrowth
enjuagar(se)	to rinse
enojado(a)	angry
enojar(se)	to anger
el enojo	anger
enrojecido(a)	reddened
el enrojecimiento	redness
enrollar(se)	to roll up
el ensanchamiento de los senos	breast enlargement
entre	between
entregar	to deliver
la envoltura	wrapper
la epiglotis	epiglottis
la EPOC (enfermedad pulmonar obstructiva crónica)	COPD (chronic obstructive pulmonary disease)
equivocado(a)	wrong, mistaken
eructar	to burp
la escala	rating scale
el escalofrío	chills
las escamas	scales (skin)
escoger	to choose
el escroto	scrotum
escuchar	to listen
escupir	to spit
esofágico(a)	esophageal
el esófago	esophagus
la esofaguitis	esophagitis
la espalda	back
esperar	to wait
espeso(a)	thick
la espinilla	pimple
la espora	spore
el espray	spray (nasal, topical)
la estación	season
el estacionamiento	parking lot
el estante	rack, stand
estar	to be (temporary)
estar(se) quieto	to stay still
la estatura	height
el estent coronario	coronary stent
el esternón	sternum, breast bone
el estetoscopio	stethoscope
estimular	to stimulate
el estómago	stomach
estornudar	to sneeze
el estornudo	sneeze
el estreñimiento	constipation
el estrés	stress
la etiqueta	label
la evacuación	bowel movement
evitar	to avoid

el excremento	excrement, stools
exhalar	to exhale, to breathe out
el expectorante	expectorant
la experiencia	experience
explicar	to explain
extender	to extend
el exterior	exterior
la extracción	extraction
facilitar	to facilitate
la falta de aliento	shortness of breath
faltar	to be lacking
febrero	February
la febrícula	low-grade fever
la fecha de caducidad, la fecha de vencimiento	expiration date
la fibra	fiber
fiebre de heno	hay fever
el (los) fín(es) de semana	weekend(s)
la flema	phlegm
flojo(a)	loose (cough), thin, lazy
fluir	to flow
el flujo	vaginal discharge
la forma	form
la formulación	formulation (chemical)
las fosas nasales	nostrils
el frasco	vial, small bottle
el frasco ámpula	injectable vial
la frecuencia	frequency
la frente	forehead
frío(a)	cold
la frustración	frustration
frustrado(a)	frustrated
frustrar(se)	to frustrate
la fruta	fruit
el fuego en la boca	mouth sore
fuerte	strong
la fuerza	force, strength
fumar	to smoke
funcionar	to function
las gafas	eyeglasses
la galleta salada	salted cracker
el galón	gallon
el ganglio, nódulo linfático	lymph node
la garganta	throat
las gárgaras	gargles
la gasa	gauze
el gel	gel
generalmente	generally
los genitales femeninos	female genitals
los genitales masculinos	male genitals
girar	to roll, to rotate
el glaucoma	glaucoma

el glucómetro	glucometer
los glúteos	buttocks
la gorra	cap (baseball)
la gota	drop
el gotero	dropper
el grado	degree
el grado centígrado	centigrade
el grado fahrenheit	Fahrenheit
el gramo	gram
grande	big
el(los) grano(s)	bump(s), little growth(s)
la grasa	fat
grasoso(a)	oily
la grieta	cracked skin
la gripe	influenza
guardar silencio	to be quiet
gustar	to like
haber (auxiliary)	to have
el hábito	habit
hablar	to talk
hacer	to do, to make
hacer ejercicio	to exercise
hacia	toward
haga buches	swish
hágalo	do it
el hambre	hunger
hay (impersonal)	there is, there are
la heces fecales	stools
la hepatitis	hepatitis
la herida	wound
el herpes genital	genital herpes
el herpes zoster	shingles
la hiedra venenosa	poison ivy (plant)
la hierba	herb
el hierro	iron
el hígado	liver
la hija	daughter
el hijo	son
hinchado(a)	swollen
la hinchazón	swelling
la hiperglicemia, la hiperglucemia	hyperglycemia
la hipertensión	hypertension
el hipo	hiccups
la hipoglicemia, la hipoglucemia	hypoglycemia
la histerectomía	hysterectomy
el (los) hombro(s)	shoulder(s)
el hongo	fungus
la hora	hour
hormiguear	to tingle (like ants)
el hormigueo	tingling (like ants)
el hueso	bone
humedecer	to moisten, to wet
húmedo(a)	damp, wet
el humo	smoke
humo de segunda mano	secondhand smoke
igual	equal, same
el impétigo	impetigo

inclinar(se)	to tilt, to lean
la incomodidad	discomfort
incómodo(a)	uncomfortable
la indigestión	indigestion
la infección	infections
la infección bucal por hongos	oral thrush
infectado(a)	infected
la inflamación	inflammation
la inflamación abdominal	bloating
inflamado(a)	inflamed
la influenza	influenza
la influenzae haemophilus tipo B	Haemophilus influenzae type B
la inhalación	inhalation, puff
el inhalador	inhaler (nasal, oral)
inhalar	to inhale
inmediatamente	immediately
la inmunización	immunization
el insomnio	insomnia
inspirar	to inhale, to inspire
la insuficiencia cardíaca congestiva	congestive heart failure
la insulina	insulin
intenso(a)	intense
el intestino delgado	small intestine
el intestino grueso	large intestine
los intestinos	intestines, bowels
la intoxicación con hiedra	poison ivy (problem)
introducir	to insert
el invierno	winter
la inyección intramuscular	intramuscular injection
la inyección intravenosa	intravenous injection
la inyección subcutánea	subcutaneous injection
inyectar(se)	to inject
ir	to go
el iris	iris
irregular	irregular
la irritabilidad	irritability
irritable	irritable
la irritación	irritation
irritado(a)	irritated
la izquierda	left
izquierdo(a)	left
el jabón	soap
jalar(se)	to pull
la jaqueca	migraine
el jarabe	syrup
la jeringa	syringe
el juanete	bunion
el jueves	Thursday
el jugo	juice

julio	July	manejar	to drive	la mudez	muteness
junio	June	la mano	hand	el mudo(a)	mute
justo	just (exactly)	mantener(se)	to keep, to stay (oneself)	muerto(a)	dead
el kilogramo	kilogram			la muñeca	wrist
los labios	lips	el maquillaje	makeup	el músculo	muscle
el lado	side	el marcapasos	pacemaker	el muslo	thigh
la lagañas	"sleep" in the eye	mareado(a)	dizzy, seasick	muy	very
el lagrimal	tearduct	el mareo	dizziness, nausea	nada	nothing
la laringe	larynx	el martes	Tuesday	las nalgas	buttocks
latir	to beat	marzo	March	la nariz	nose
lavar(se)	to wash with soap	la mascota	pet	la nariz tapada	congested nose
		masticable	chewable	la náusea	nausea
el laxante	laxative	masticar	to chew	necesitar	to need
la leche	milk	matar	to kill	negro(a)	black
la legumbres	legumes	la matriz	uterus	el nerviosismo	nervousness
la lengua	tongue	mayo	May	nervioso(a)	nervous
la lengüeta de la oreja	tragus, "earflap"	la medida	measurement	la neumonía	pneumonia
		el medidor de aliento, flujo máximo pulmonar	peak flow meter	la neuropatía	neuropathy
lentamente	slowly			neutralizar	to neutralize
los lentes	eyeglasses	el medio ambiente	environment	la niña	girl
lento(a)	slow	medir	to measure	el niño	boy
la lesión	lesion	las mejillas	cheeks	el nivel	level
levantar(se)	to stand up/get up	mejor	better	normal	normal
leve	slight	mejorar(se)	to feel better	notar	to notice
la libra	pound	el meningocócico	meningococcal	noviembre	November
la licencia de manejar, la licencia de conducir	drivers license	la menopausia	menopause	la nuca	nape
		menor	minor	nunca	never
		la menstruación	menstruation	nunca jamás	never ever
ligeramente	slightly, lightly	la menta	mint	o	or
ligero(a)	light	el mentón	chin	o sea	in other words
limpiar(se)	to clean	el mes	month	observar	to observe, to watch
limpio (a)	clean	el metro	meter		
la línea	line	la mezcla	mixture	la obstrucción intestinal	intestinal obstruction
el líquido	liquid	mezclar	to mix		
líquido(a)	runny	el mezquino	wart	octubre	October
el litro	liter	el miembro	member (penis)	ocupado(a)	busy
la llaga	sore	mientras	while	la oficina	office
llamar(se)	to name, to call	el miércoles	Wednesday	el oftalmólogo	ophthalmologist
llenar	to fill with a volume	la migraña	migraine	el oído de nadador	swimmer's ear
		el miligramo	milligram	el (los) oído(s)	inner ear(s)
llevar	to take, to carry	el mililitro	milliliter	oir	to hear
llorar	to cry	el minuto	minute	el (los) ojo(s)	eye(s)
lloroso(a)	tearful, weeping	mirar	to look	oler	to smell
el lóbulo de la oreja	ear lobe	el moco	mucus	el olor	odor, smell
la loción	lotion (facial), cologne, clear solutions	el moho	mold, mildew	olvidar(se)	to forget
		mojado(a)	wet	el ombligo	navel
		la molestia	discomfort	la onza	ounce
la loción limpiadora	cleanser	molesto(a)	bothersome	opaco(a)	opaque
la loción para después de rasurarse (afeitarse)	after-shave lotion	el momento	moment	la opresión en el pecho	chest tightness
		morado(a)	purple	oprimir(se)	to press
luego	later	morder	to bite	oral	oral
el lunar	mole	el moretón	bruise	la(s) oreja(s)	outer ear(s)
el lunes	Monday	morir	to die	los órganos	organs
la luz (las luces)	light(s)	el mostrador	counter	el orificio	orifice, opening
el magnesio	magnesium	mostrar	to show	la orina	urine
mal	bad	mover(se)	to move	orinar	to urinate
el malestar	discomfort	muchísimo(a)	very much	el orzuelo	stye
el malparto	miscarriage	mucho(a)	a lot, much	oscuro(a)	dark
manchado(a)	spotted	la mucosa	mucus (membrane)	la otitis media	otitis media
mandar	to send			el otoño	autumn

el otorrinolaringó-logo(a)	ear, nose, and throat doctor	la pestaña	eyelash
el otoscopio	otoscope	el pezón	nipple
otra vez	again	la picadura de abeja	bee sting
el ovario	ovary	picante	hot, spicy
el óvulo vaginal	vaginal suppository	picar(se)	to pinch
el paciente asmático	asthmatic patient	la picazón	intense itching, prickling
el país	country	el pie de atleta	athlete's foot
la palabra	word	el pie	foot
pálido(a)	pale	la piel	skin
la palma de la mano	palm (hand)	la pierna	leg
palpar	to palpate	la píldora	very small round pills, "the pill"
la palpitación	palpitation, throbbing	la pinta	pint
el pan integral	whole-grain bread	la pipí (euphemism)	urine
el páncreas	pancreas	el piquete	stick, bite
la pantorrilla	calf	el piquete de mosquito	mosquito bite
el papanicolau	Pap smear	el piso	floor
el papel higénico, sanitario	toilet paper	plano(a)	dull
las papilas gustativas	taste buds	la planta	plant
parar(se)	to stand	la planta del pie	sole
el parche	patch	plástico(a)	plastic
la pared	wall	poco(a)	little
parpadear	to blink	poder	to be able to (can)
el(los) párpado(s)	eyelid(s)	el polen	pollen
la parte	part	la poliomielitis, la polio	polio
las partes privadas, los genitales	private parts, genitals	el polvo	medicinal powder (often oral), dust
pasar	to pass through	la pomada	ointment, cream
pasar de	to be over	las pompis (euphemism)	buttocks
el pasillo	aisle	el pómulo(s)	cheekbone(s)
la pastilla	pill	poner(se)	to place, to put
las pecas	freckles	la popó (euphemism)	feces, stools
el pecho	chest (breast)	por dentro	inside
pedir	to order	por eso	for that reason
peinar(se)	to comb	por lo menos	at least
el peine	comb	la porción	portion
peligroso(a)	dangerous	el precio	price
pellizcar(se)	to pinch	preferir	to prefer
el pelo	hair	preocupar(se)	to worry
la pelvis	pelvis	la presentación	formulation (packaged)
el pene	penis	la presión	pressure
pensar	to think	la presión alta	high blood pressure
peor	worse	la presión arterial	blood pressure
pequeño(a)	small, little	prevenir	to prevent, to avoid
perder	to lose	la primavera	spring
la pérdida	loss	el principio	the beginning
la pérdida del oído	hearing loss	el problema	problem
el perfume	perfume	producir	to produce
el período	menstruation, period	el producto	product
la perla	soft gel capsule	profundo(a)	deep
permanecer	to keep, to stay	pronto	soon
la perrilla	stye	propio(a)	your own
persistente	persistent	la próstata	prostate
pesar	to weigh		
el peso	weight		

el protector solar	sunscreen
proteger	to protect
provocar	to provoke
la prueba de esfuerzo	stress test
el prurito de los jockeys	jock itch
el puente coronario	coronary bypass
la puerta	door
la pulgada	inch
el (los) pulmón(es)	lung(s)
pulmonar	pulmonary
la pulmonía	pneumonia
la pulsación	pulsation
el pulso	pulse
el punto blanco	whitehead
el punto negro	blackhead
la punzada	sharp pain
la punzada de oído	earache
la pupila	pupil
el purgante	purgative
la pus	pus
quejar(se)	to complain
la quemadura	burn
la quemadura de sol	sunburn
quemar(se)	to burn
querer	to want
quitar(se)	to get rid of, to take off
rápido(a)	rapid, fast
rascar(se)	to scratch
la raspadura	scratch
el raspón	scratch
rasurar(se)	to shave
la reacción	reaction
el recibo	receipt
recoger	to pick up
recomendar	to recommend
rectal	rectal
redondo(a)	circular, round
el reembolso	refund
el reflujo	reflux
el refresco	soft drink
refrigerar	to refrigerate
el refuerzo	booster
regir	to move the bowels
la regla	menstruation
regresar	to return
regular	regular
relajar(se)	to relax
remangar	to roll up sleeves
remojar	to soak
repetir	to repeat, to belch
reponer	to replace
la resaca	hangover
resecar	to dry out
reseco(a)	dry
la resequedad	dryness
el resfrío	cold

Spanish	English
la(s) respiración(es)	breath(s), respiration(s)
respirar	to breathe
resurtir	to refill
retirar	to take away, to take out
revisar(se)	to check, to revise (oneself)
la rigidez	stiffness
El (los) riñón(es)	kidney(s)
el rocío	sprinkle, aerosol
la rodilla	knee
rojo(a)	red
romper	to break, to tear
la roña	scabies (common)
las ronchas	hives
la ropa	clothes
la ropa de cama	bed linens
rosa	pink
la rozadura de pañal	diaper rash
la rubéola	rubella
el ruido	noise
el sábado	Saturday
saber	to know
sabor a cereza	cherry-flavored
sabor a frutas	fruit-flavored
el sabor a pimienta	peppery taste
sabor a uva	grape-flavored
sacar	to take out
la sal	salt
salir	to go out, to leave
el salpullido	rash
las sandalias	sandals
sangrar	to bleed
la sangre	blood
el sarampión	measles
la sarna	scabies (technical)
el sarpullido	rash
secar(se)	to dry
seco(a)	dry
la sed	thirst
seguir	to follow, to continue
el segundo	second
seguro(a)	safe (for use), certain
el seguro	insurance
el sello	seal
la semana	week
la señal	sign
el seno, el pecho	breast
los senos nasales	nasal sinuses
la sensación	sensation
sensibilidad	sensitivity
sentar(se)	to sit
el sentimiento de soledad	loneliness
sentir(se)	to feel
septiembre	September
ser	to be (permanent)
servir(se)	to serve, to help
el SIDA (síndrome de inmunodeficiencia adquirida)	AIDS (acquired immunodeficiency syndrome)
siempre	always
la(s) sien(es)	temple(s)
el signo	sign
el silbido	wheezing
la silla	chair
simple	simple
sin	without
síndrome de abstinencia	withdrawal
el síntoma	symptom
la sinusitis	sinusitis
el sobrante	excess
sobrepeso	overweight
sólido(a)	thick, solid
sólo, solamente	only
soltar	to release
la soltura	diarrhea
la solución	solution
el sombrero	hat
la somnolencia	drowsiness (from medicine, disease)
sonar(se)	to blow one's nose
soplar	to blow out
el soplo	murmur (heart)
la sordera	deafness
sordo(a)	dull (pain), mute
suavemente	gently
suavizar	to soften
el suelo	floor
el sueño	sleepiness, dream
el suero	intravenous mixtures
el suero oral	oral rehydration solution
sufrir	to suffer
el supositorio	suppository
la supuración	oozing, suppuration
supurar	to suppurate (pus), to ooze
surtir	to fill (an order)
la suspensión	suspension
la suspensión coloide	colloid suspension
la tableta	tablet
el talco	talc, powder (skin)
el talón	heel
también	too, also
el tampón	tampon
la tapa	lid
tardar	to take time
la tarjeta de crédito	credit card
la tarjeta de seguro	insurance card
la taza	cup
la temperatura	temperature
temporalmente	temporarily
tener	to have
tener ganas	to feel like, to have the urge
tener que	to have to
la tensión	tension
tenso(a)	tense
terco(a)	stubborn
el termómetro	thermometer
el testículo	testicle
el tétanos	tetanus
tibio(a)	lukewarm
el tiempo	time
el timbre	bell
el tímpano	eardrum, tympannic membrane
el tinnitus	tinnitus (ringing)
el tipo	type
la tira	strip
tirar	to dispose
la tiroides	thyroid
la toalla sanitaria	sanitary pad
el tobillo	ankle
tocar	to touch
todavía	still
tolerable	tolerable
tomar	to take, to drink
tópico(a)	topical
los toques	medication for mouth applied in "touches"
la tos	cough
toser	to cough
la tosferina	pertussis
la toxicidad	toxicity
tragar	to swallow
transparente	clear, transparent
la tráquea	trachea
el trasplante de corazón	heart transplant
el tratamiento	treatment
tratar	to try, to treat (illness)
tricúspide	tricuspid
triste	sad
la tristeza	sadness
el trocisco	troche
las trompas de Falopio	fallopian tubes
la tuberculosis	tuberculosis
el tubo	tube
el tubo de extensión	"spacer"
turístico(a)	tourist-like
la úlcera	ulcer
últimamente	lately

la uña enterrada	ingrown nail	el vaso	glass	el viernes	Friday
la uña	fingernail, toenail	el vegetal	vegetable	el VIH (virus de inmunodeficiencia humana)	HIV (human immunodeficiency virus)
el ungüento	cream, ointment	el vello	body hair		
la(s) unidad(es)	unit(s)	la vena	vein		
la uretra	urethra	vencer(se)	to expire	viral (de virus)	viral
la urticaria	urticaria	el vencimiento	expiration	la viruela loca	chicken pox
usar	to use	la ventana	window	la viruela	smallpox
usualmente	usually	las ventanas nasales	nostrils	el virus del papiloma humano (VPH)	human papilloma virus (HPV)
el útero	uterus	el ventrículo	ventricle		
utilizar	to utilize	ver	to see	viscoso(a)	thick, viscous
la vacuna	immunization, vaccine, vaccination	el verano	summer	la visión borrosa	blurry vision
		verde	green	vomitar	to vomit
		verdoso(a)	greenish	el vómito	vomit
las vacunas muertas	killed vaccines	la verdura	vegetable	la vulva	vulva
las vacunas vivas	live vaccines	el vértigo	vertigo	y	and
la vagina	vagina	la vesícula biliar	gallbladder	el zapato	shoe
la válvula	valve	las vesículas seminales	seminal vesicles	la zona (verde, amarilla, roja)	zone (green, yellow, red)
la varicela	chicken pox				
la vaselina	Vaseline®, petroleum jelly	viajar	to travel	el zumbido	ringing
		las vías respiratorias	airway passages		
		el vientre	abdomen		

Glosario inglés–español
English–Spanish glossary

a lot of, too much	demasiado(a)	allergy	la alergia
a lot, much	mucho(a)	to alleviate	aliviar
abdomen	el abdomen, el vientre	aluminum	el aluminio
		always	siempre
abdominal cramp	el cólico	ampule	la ampolleta
abdominal tension	la distensión dis- abdominal	amputation	la amputación
		analgesic	el analgésico
abdominal pain	el dolor abdominal	and	y, e
abortion (induced)	el aborto provocado	anesthetic	el anestésico
		anger	el enojo
above	arriba	to anger	enojar(se)
acid	ácido(a)	angina	la angina
acidity	las acedías, las agruras	angioplasty	la angioplastía
		angry	enojado(a)
acne	el acné	animal dander	la caspa animal
across, through	a través	ankle	el tobillo
addiction	la adicción	antacid	el antiácido
adult	el adulto, la adulta	antibacterial	el antibacteriano
to affect	afectar(se)	antihistamine	el antihistamínico
affected	afectado(a)	antiseptic	el antiséptico
after, later	después (de)	anxiety	la ansiedad
after-shave lotion	la loción para después de rasurarse (afeitarse)	aortic	aórtica
		apparatus, device	el aparato
		appetite	el apetito
		applicator	el aplicador
again	otra vez	to apply, to instill	aplicar(se)
age	la edad	April	abril
AIDS (acquired immunodeficiency syndrome)	el SIDA (sín drome de inmunodeficien- cia adquirida)	arch of the foot	el arco del pie
		area	el área
		arm	el brazo
		around	alrededor
air	el aire	artery	la arteria
airway passages	las vías respiratorias	asthma	el asma
aisle	el pasillo	asthma attack	el ataque de asma
alcoholic	alcohólico(a)	at least	por lo menos
allergen	el alérgeno	atherosclerosis	la aterosclerosis
allergic	alérgico(a)	athlete's foot	el pie de atleta

atrium	la aurícula
to attach	conectar
August	agosto
aura	el aura
auscultation	la auscultación
autumn	el otoño
to avoid	evitar
axillary	la axila
back	atrás
back (anatomical)	la espalda
back of hand	el dorso de la mano
backward, opposite side	al revés
bacteria	la bacteria
bad	mal
bag	la bolsa
bandage	el curita
barrel (of inhaler)	el barril
bathroom	el baño
to be (permanent)	ser
to be (temporary)	estar
to be able to (can)	poder
to be certain	asegurar(se)
to be lacking	faltar
to be over	pasar de
to be quiet	guardar silencio
to beat	latir
bed linens	la ropa de cama
bee sting	la picadura de abeja
before	antes (de)
to begin	comenzar, empezar
beginning	el principio
to believe	creer
bell	la campanilla, el timbre
below	debajo
to bend over	agachar(se)

better	mejor	buttocks	las asentaderas, los glúteos, las nalgas, las pompis (euphemism)	clear	claro(a), transparente
between	entre			clear broth	el caldo
bicuspid or mitral	bicúspide o mitral			clogged arteries	las arterias obstruidas
big	grande	bypass	la cirugía de derivación coronaria		
to bite	morder			to close	cerrar
bitter	amargo(a)			closed	cerrado(a)
black	negro(a)	caffeine	la cafeína	clot	el coágulo
blackhead	el barro, el punto negro	calcium	el calcio	clothes	la ropa
		calf	la pantorrilla	coat	el abrigo
to bleed	sangrar	cap (baseball)	la cachucha, la gorra	cold	frío(a)
blind	ciego(a)			cold (illness)	el resfrío
blindness	la ceguera	capsule	la cápsula	colloid suspension	la suspensión coloide
to blink	parpadear	cardiac catheterization	cateterismo cardíaco		
blister	la ampolla			color	el color
bloating	la inflamación abdominal	cardiologist	el cardiólogo, la cardióloga	comb	el peine
				to comb	peinar(se)
blood	la sangre	case (situation)	el caso	comfort, well-being	el bienestar
blood pressure	la presión arterial	cash	el efectivo	common	común
blood pressure cuff	el brazalete del baumanómetro	cash register	la caja	to complain	quejar(se)
		cashier's desk	la caja registradora	computer	la computadora
to blow one's nose	sonar(se)	cause	la causa	to confirm	confirmar
to blow out	soplar	to cause	causar	confuse	confuso(a)
blue	azul	Celsius	el grado centígrado	confusion	la confusión
blurry	borroso(a)	centimeter	el centímetro	congested nose	la nariz tapada, congestionada
body	el cuerpo	cents	los centavos		
body hair	el vello	cervix	el cervix	conjunctivitis	la conjuntivitis
bone	el hueso	chair	la silla	consistency	la consistencia
booster	el refuerzo, el búster (popular)	change	el cambio	constipation	el estreñimiento
		to change	cambiar(se)	to consult	consultar
bothersome	molesto(a)	to charge	cargar	to contain	contener
bottle	la botella	check	el cheque	to contaminate, to get infected	contagiar(se)
bottle, vial	el frasco	to check oneself	checar(se), revisar(se)		
bowel movement	la evacuación			continuous	continuo(a)
boy	el niño	cheekbone	el pómulo	to contract, to acquire a disease	contraer
brain	el cerebro	cheeks	las mejillas		
to break, to tear	romper	cherry-flavored	sabor a cereza	to control	controlar
breakfast	el desayuno	chest	el pecho	COPD (chronic obstructive pulmonary disease)	la EPOC (enfermedad pulmonar obstructiva crónica)
breast	el seno, el pecho	chest congestion	la congestión del pecho		
breast enlargement	el ensanchamiento de los senos				
		chest tightness	la opresión en el pecho	corn, callus	el callo
breast tenderness	los senos adoloridos			coronary bypass	el puente coronario
		to chew	masticar	correct	correcto(a)
breath, air in lungs	el aliento	chewable	masticable	cotton	el algodón
breath, respiration	la respiración	chicken pox	la viruela loca, la varicela	cough	la tos
to breathe	respirar			to cough	toser
bright	brillante	chills	el escalofrío	counter	el mostrador
bronchi	los bronquios	chin	la barbilla, el mentón	country	el país
bronchitis	la bronquitis			coupon	el cupón
brown	café	to choose	escoger	to cover	cubrir(se)
bruise	el moretón	chronic illness	la enfermedad crónica	cracked (skin)	la grieta
brush	el cepillo			cracker (salted)	la galleta salada
bubble	la burbuja	chrysanthemum	el crisantemo	cramp	el calambre
bumps (little growths)	los granos	circular	redondo(a)	cream, lotion	la crema
bunion	el juanete	circulation	la circulación	cream, ointment	el ungüento, la pomada
burn	la quemadura	clean	limpio(a)		
to burn	arder(se), quemar(se)	to clean	limpiar(se)	credit card	la tarjeta de crédito
		cleanser	la loción limpiadora	to cry	llorar
to burp	eructar			cup	la taza
busy	ocupado(a)				

to cure	curar(se)
currently	actualmente
cut	la cortada, la cortadura
cyanosis	la cianosis
cyanotic	cianótico(a)
cycle	el ciclo
damaging	dañino(a)
damp	húmedo(a)
dandruff	la caspa
dangerous	peligroso(a)
dark	oscuro(a)
daughter	la hija
day	el día
dead	muerto(a)
deafness	la sordera
December	diciembre
deep	profundo(a)
degree	el grado
to deliver	entregar
deodorant	el desodorante
to deposit	depositar
depressed	deprimido(a)
depression	la depresión
dermatitis	la dermatitis
to describe	describir
device	el dispositivo
diaper rash	la rozadura de pañal
diarrhea	la diarrea, la soltura
to die	morir
different	diferente
difficulty	la dificultad
difficulty breathing	dificultad para respirar
dinner, evening meal	la cena
diphtheria	la difteria
directly	directamente
discharge	el desecho
discomfort	la incomodidad, el malestar, la molestia
to disinfect	desinfectar
disposable	desechable
to dispose	tirar
to dissolve	disolver
dizziness, nausea	el mareo
dizzy, seasick	mareado(a)
to do, to make	hacer
door	la puerta
dose(s)	la dosis (las dosis)
douche (feminine)	la ducha femenina
down, below	abajo
drawer	el cajón
drink	la bebida
to drink	beber
to drive	manejar
driver's license	la licencia de manejar, la licencia de conducir

drop	la gota
dropper	el gotero
drowsiness (from medicine or disease)	la somnolencia
drunk	borracho(a) (slang)
drunkenness	la ebriedad, borrachera (slang)
dry	reseco(a), seco(a)
to dry	secar(se)
to dry out	resecar
dryness	la resequedad
dull	plano(a), sordo(a)
during	durante
dust	el polvo
dust mites	los ácaros del polvo
each, every	cada
ear (inner)	el oído
ear (outer)	la oreja
ear lobe	el lóbulo de la oreja
ear, nose, and throat doctor	el (la) otorrinolaringólogo(a)
earache	la punzada de oído
eardrum	el tímpano
earwax	la cerilla, el cerumen
to eat	comer
echocardiogram	la ecocardiografía
effective	efectivo(a)
effervescent	efervescente
elbow	el codo
electrolyte replacement	el suero oral
electrocardiogram, EKG	el electrocardiograma
elevator	el ascensor, el elevador
elixir	el elíxir
emergency	la emergencia
emotional	emotivo(a)
emphysema	el enfisema pulmonar
emulsion	la emulsión
end of the line	la cola
enema	el enema
enlargement	el agrandamiento
enteral feeding	la alimentación por sonda
environment	el medio ambiente
epiglottis	la epiglotis
equal, same	igual
erectile dysfunction	la disfunción eréctil
esophageal	esofágico(a)
esophagitis	la esofaguitis
esophagus	el esófago
every day	diariamente
excess	el sobrante
excrement, stool	el excremento

to excuse, to be sorry	disculpar
exercise	el ejercicio
to exercise	hacer ejercicio
to exhale, to breathe out	exhalar
expectorant	el expectorante
expensive	caro(a)
experience	la experiencia
expiration	la caducidad, el vencimiento
to expire	caducar, vencer(se)
to explain	explicar
to extend	extender
exterior	el exterior
extraction	la extracción
eye	el ojo
eyebrow	la ceja
eyeglasses	los anteojos, las gafas, los lentes
eyelash	la pestaña
eyelid	el párpado
face	la cara
to facilitate	facilitar
Fahrenheit	el grado fahrenheit
fainting	el desvanecimiento
fall (season)	el otoño
fallopian tubes	las trompas de Falopio
fat	la grasa
fatigue	el cansancio
February	febrero
feces, stools	la popó (euphemism)
to feel	sentir(se)
to feel better	aliviar(se) / mejorar(se)
to feel like, to have an urge	tener ganas
feminine genitals	los genitales femeninos
fever	la calentura
fiber	la fibra
to fill (an order)	surtir
to fill (with a volume)	llenar
finger cot (rubber)	el dedal de hule
fingers	los dedos de la mano
floor	el piso, el suelo
to flow	fluir
to follow, to continue	seguir
food	la comida
foot	el pie
for example	por ejemplo
for that reason	por eso
force, strength	la fuerza
forearm	el antebrazo
forehead	la frente
to forget	olvidar(se)
form	la forma

formulation (chemical)	la formulación
formulation (packaged)	la presentación
freckles	las pecas
frequency	la frecuencia
Friday	el viernes
fruit	la fruta
fruit-flavored	sabor a frutas
to frustrate	frustrar(se)
frustrated	frustrado(a)
frustration	la frustración
to function	funcionar
fungus	el hongo
fungus of the mouth	el hongo de la boca
gallbladder	la vesícula biliar
gallon	el galón
gargles	las gárgaras
garlic	el ajo
gauze	la gasa
gel	el gel
generally	generalmente
genital herpes	el herpes genital
gently	suavemente
to get rid of, to take off	quitar(se)
girl	la niña
to give	dar
glass	el vaso
glaucoma	el glaucoma
glucometer	el glucómetro
to go	ir
to go down, to lower	bajar
to go out, to leave	salir
gram	el gramo
grape-flavored	sabor a uva
green	verde
greenish	verdoso(a)
gum (chewing)	el chicle
gums	las encías
habit	el hábito
Haemophilus influenzae type B	la influenzae haemophilus tipo B
hair	el cabello, el pelo
hand	la mano
hangover	la resaca, la cruda (slang)
hard	duro(a)
to harden	endurecer
harmful	dañino(a)
hat	el sombrero
to have	haber (auxiliary)
to have	tener
to have to	tener que
hay fever	fiebre de heno
head	la cabeza
to hear	oír
hearing loss	la pérdida del oído
heart	el corazón

heart attack	el ataque cardiaco, el ataque al corazón
heart failure (congestive)	la insuficiencia cardíaca congestiva
heart transplant	el trasplante de corazón
heartburn	la acidez
to heat, to warm	calentar
heel	el talón
height	la estatura
helmet	el casco
to help	ayudar
help, support	el apoyo
hepatitis	la hepatitis
herb	la hierba
hiccups	el hipo
high	alto(a)
high blood pressure	la presión alta
high cholesterol	el colesterol alto
hip	la cadera
HIV (human immuno-deficiency virus)	el VIH (virus de inmunodeficien-cia humana)
hives	las ronchas
hold the breath	contener la respiración
hot, spicy	picante
hot, warm	caliente
hot flashes	los bochornos
hour	la hora
human papilloma virus (HPV)	el virus del papi-loma humano (VPH)
hunger	el hambre
to hurt, to be in pain	doler(se)
hyperglycemia	la hiperglicemia, la hiperglucemia
hypertension	la hipertensión
hypoglycemia	la hipoglicemia, la hipoglucemia
hysterectomy	la histerectomía
immediately	inmediatamente
immunization	la inmunización, la vacuna
impetigo	el impétigo
in front	(en)frente
in other words	o sea
inch	la pulgada
indigestion	la indigestión
inexpensive	barato(a)
infected	infectado(a)
infection	la infección
inflamed	inflamado(a)
inflammation	la inflamación
influenza	la gripe, la influenza
ingrown toenail	la uña enterrada
inhalation, puff	la inhalación

to inhale	inhalar
to inhale, to inspire	inspirar
inhaler (nasal, oral)	el inhalador
to inject	inyectar(se)
injectable vial	el frasco ámpula
inner ear	el oído
to insert	introducir
inside	(a)dentro
inside	por dentro
insomnia	el insomnio
insulin	la insulina
insurance card	la tarjeta de seguro
intense	intenso(a)
intense itching	la picazón
intestinal obstruction	la obstrucción intestinal
intestine(s), bowel(s)	el intestino (los intestinos)
intramuscular injection	la inyección intramuscular
intravenous injection	la inyección intravenosa
intravenous mixtures	el suero
iris	el iris
iron	el hierro
irregular	irregular
irritability	la irritabilidad
irritable	irritable
irritated	irritado(a)
irritation	la irritación
itchiness	la comezón
itchiness (stronger)	la picazón
item	el artículo
January	enero
jock itch	el prurito de los jockeys
joint	la articulación
juice	el jugo
July	julio
June	junio
just (exactly)	justo
to keep, to stay	permanecer
to keep, to stay	mantener(se)
kidney(s)	el riñón (los riñones)
to kill	matar
killed vaccines	las vacunas muertas
kilogram	el kilogramo
knee	la rodilla
knee-highs	las calcetas
to know	saber
label	la etiqueta
lack of sensation in the feet	la falta de sensibil-idad en los pies
large intestine	el intestino grueso
larynx	la laringe
lately	últimamente
later	luego
laxative	el laxante

layer	la capa	menstruation	la menstruación, la regla, el período	to notice	notar
leap year	el año bisiesto			November	noviembre
left	la izquierda	meter	el metro	now	ahora
left	izquierdo(a)	migraine	la jaqueca, la migraña	oatmeal	la avena
leg	la pierna			to observe	observar
legumes	las legumbres	milk	la leche	October	octubre
lesion	la lesión	milligram	el miligramo	office	la oficina
level	el nivel	milliliter	el mililitro	oil	el aceite
lid	la tapa	minor	menor	oily	grasoso(a)
to lie down, to go to bed	acostar(se)	mint	la menta	ointment, cream	la pomada, el ungüento
		minute	el minuto		
light (not heavy)	ligero(a)	miscarriage	el aborto natural, el malparto	on your back or face up	boca arriba
light(s)	la luz (las luces)				
to like	gustar	to mix	mezclar	on your side	de lado
line	la línea	mixture	la mezcla	onion	la cebolla
lips	los labios	to moisten, to wet	humedecer	only	sólo, solamente
liquid	el líquido	mold, mildew	el moho	oozing	la supuración
to listen	escuchar	mole	el lunar	opaque	opaco(a)
liter	el litro	moment	el momento	to open	abrir(se)
little	chico(a), pequeño(a), poco(a)	Monday	el lunes	ophthalmologist	el oftalmólogo
		money	el dinero	or	o, u
		month	el mes	oral	oral
live vaccines	las vacunas vivas	more than	más de, más que	oral rehydration solution	el suero oral
liver	el hígado	mosquito bite	el piquete de mosquito		
loneliness	el sentimiento de soledad			oral thrush	la infección bucal por hongos
		mouth	la boca		
to look	mirar	mouth sores	el fuego en la boca	oral thrush (cotton-like)	el algodoncillo (slang)
loose (cough)	flojo(a)	to move the bowels	regir		
to lose	perder	to move	mover(se)	orange	anaranjado(a)
to lose weight	bajar de peso	mucus	el moco, la mucosa	to order	pedir
loss	la pérdida	mumps	las paperas	organs	los órganos
lotion (facial), cologne	la loción	murmur	el soplo	orifice, opening	el orificio
		muscle	el músculo	otitis media	la otitis media
low-grade fever	la febrícula	mute (person)	el (la) mudo(a), el (la) sordo(a)	otoscope	el otoscopio
lukewarm	tibio(a)			ounce	la onza
lukewarm water	el agua tibia	muteness	la mudez	out of reach	fuera del alcance
lung(s)	el pulmón (los pulmones)	nail	la uña	outer ear	la oreja
		to name, to call	llamar(se)	outside	afuera
lying with your face down	boca abajo	nape	la nuca	ovary	el ovario
		nasal congestion	la congestión nasal	overgrowth	el engrosamiento
lymph node	el ganglio, nódulo linfático	nasal sinuses	los senos nasales	overweight	sobrepeso
		nausea	el asco, la náusea	pacemaker	el marcapasos
magnesium	el magnesio	navel	el ombligo	pain	el dolor
makeup	el maquillaje	neck	el cuello	pale	pálido(a)
March	marzo	to need	necesitar	palm	la palma
masculine genitals	los genitales masculinos	needle	la aguja	palpitation, throbbing	la palpitación
		nervous	nervioso(a)	to palpate	palpar
May	mayo	nervousness	el nerviosismo	pancreas	el páncreas
meal	la comida	neuropathy	la neuropatía	Pap smear	el papanicolau
measles	el sarampión	to neutralize	neutralizar	parking lot	el estacionamiento
to measure	medir	never	nunca	part	la parte
measurement	la medida	never ever	nunca jamás	to pass through (e.g., stomach)	pasar
medication for the mouth (applied in "touches")	los toques	nipple	el pezón		
		noise	el ruido	patch	el parche
		normal	normal	peak flow meter	el medidor de aliento, el flujo máximo pulmonar
		nose	la nariz		
medicinal powder (often oral)	el polvo	nostrils	las fosas nasales, las ventanas nasales		
meningococcal	el meningocócico			to peel (skin)	despellejar
menopause	la menopausia	no more	nada más	pelvis	la pelvis

penis	el pene (el miembro)	quart	el cuarto de galón	season	la estación
peppery taste	el sabor a pimienta	quit smoking	dejar de fumar	second	el segundo
perfume	el perfume	rack, stand	el estante	secondhand smoke	el humo de
to permit, to allow, to leave	dejar	rapid, fast	rápido(a)		segunda mano
		rash	el sarpullido,	to see	ver
persistent	persistente		el salpullido	seminal vesicles	las vesículas
pertussis	la tosferina	rating scale	la escala		seminales
pet	la mascota	reaction	la reacción	to send	mandar
phlegm	la flema	receipt	el recibo	sensation	la sensación
to pick up	recoger	to recommend	recomendar	sensitivity	sensibilidad
pill	la pastilla,	rectal	rectal	September	septiembre
	el comprimido	red	rojo(a)	to serve, to help	servir(se)
pill (very small round), "the pill"	la píldora	reddened	enrojecido(a)	to shake	agitar
		redness	el enrojecimiento	shampoo	el champú
pimple	la espinilla	to refill	resurtir	sharp	agudo(a)
to pinch	pellizcar(se)	reflux	el reflujo	sharp pain	la punzada
pink	rosa	to refrigerate	refrigerar	to shave	rasurar(se)
pint	la pinta	refund	el reembolso	shingles	el herpes zoster
to place	colocar, poner	regular	regular	shoes	los zapatos
plant	la planta	to relax	relajar(se)	short	bajo(a)
plastic	plástico(a)	to release	soltar	shortness	la falta de aliento
plunger (applicator part)	el émbolo	to relieve	calmar(se)	of breath	
		to repeat	repetir	should, must	deber (de)
pneumonia	la neumonía,	to replace	reponer	shoulder(s)	el(los) hombro(s)
	la pulmonia	respiratory infection	la infección	to show	mostrar
poison ivy (plant)	la hiedra venenosa		respiratoria	side	el lado
poison ivy (problem)	la intoxicación con	to rest	descansar	sign	la señal
	hiedra	to return	regresar	sign	el signo
polio	la poliomielitis,	to revise, to check	revisar	simple	simple
	la polio	rib	la costilla	since yesterday	desde ayer
pollen	el polen	right (direction)	el (la) derecho(a)	sinusitis	la sinusitis
portion	la porción	right now	ahora mismo	to sit	sentar(se)
pound	la libra	ringing	el zumbido	skin	la piel
powder (skin)	el talco	to rinse	enjuagar(se)	to sleep	dormir(se)
powder, dust	el polvo	to roll, to rotate	girar	sleep, dream	el sueño
to prefer	preferir	to roll up	enrollar(se)	"sleep" in the eye	la lagañas
pregnancy	el embarazo	to roll up sleeves	remangar(se)	slight	leve
to press	oprimir(se)	room	el cuarto	slightly, lightly	ligeramente
pressure	la presión	rubella	la rubéola	slow	lento(a)
to prevent	prevenir, evitar	runny	líquido(a)	slowly	lentamente
price	el precio	runny nose	el catarro	small	chico(a),
prickling	la picazón	sad	triste		pequeño(a)
private parts, genitals	las partes privadas, los genitales	sadness	la tristeza	small device	el aparatito
		safe, reliable	confiable	small intestine	el intestino
problem	el problema	safe (for use), certain	seguro(a)		delgado
to produce	producir	salt	la sal	smallpox	la viruela
product	el producto	sandals	las sandalias	smell	el olor
prostate	la próstata	sanitary pad	la toalla sanitaria	to smell	oler
to protect	proteger	Saturday	el sábado	smoke	el humo
to provoke	provocar	to say, to tell	decir	to smoke	fumar
to pull	jalar(se)	scabies	la sarna (technical),	smoothly	suavemente
pulmonary	pulmonar		la roña	snack	el bocadillo
pulsation	la pulsación	scales (skin)	las escamas	sneeze	el estornudo
pulse	el pulso	scalp	el cuero cabelludo	to sneeze	estornudar
pupil	la pupila	scarf	la bufanda	to soak	remojar
purgative	el purgante	scratch	la raspadura, el	soap	el jabón
purple	morado(a)		raspón	socks	los calcetines
pus	la pus	to scratch	rascar(se)	sodium bicarbonate	el bicarbonato de
to push	empujar	scrotum	el escroto		sodio
quantity	la cantidad	seal	el sello	soft	blando(a)

soft drink	el refresco
soft gel capsule	la perla
to soften	suavizar
sole	la planta del pie
solution	la solución
sometimes	a veces, de vez en cuando
son	el hijo
sooner	pronto
sore	adolorido(a)
sore	la llaga
sour, acid, tart	agrio(a)
"spacer"	el tubo de extensión
sphygmomanometer, blood pressure manometer	el baumanómetro
spicy, seasoned	condimentado(a)
to spit	escupir
spore	la espora
spotted	manchado(a)
spray	el atomizador
spray (nasal, topical)	el aerosol, el espray
spray bottle	el espray
spring (season)	la primavera
sprinkle, aerosol	el rocío
to squeeze, to press	apretar
to stand	parar(se)
to stand up	levantar(se)
to stay still	estar(se) quieto
stent	el estent coronario
sternum, breast bone	el esternón
stethoscope	el estetoscopio
stick, sting, bite	el piquete
stiffness	la rigidez
still	todavía
to stimulate	estimular
to sting	picar
stomach	el estómago
stools	las heces fecales
to stop, to quit	dejar (de)
straight, straight ahead	derecho
stress	el estrés
stress test	la prueba de esfuerzo
strip	la tira
stroke	la apoplejía, la embolia, el derrame cerebral
strong	fuerte
stubborn	terca
stye	el orzuelo, la perrilla
subcutaneous injection	la inyección subcutánea
to suck on	chupar
to suffer	sufrir
sugar	el azúcar

summer	el verano
sunblock	el bloqueador de sol
sunburn	la quemadura de sol
Sunday	el domingo
sunscreen	el protector solar
suntan lotion	el bronceador
suppository	el supositorio
to suppurate (pus), to ooze	supurar
suppuration	la supuración
suspension	la suspensión
to swallow	tragar
swelling	la hinchazón
swimmer's ear	el oído de nadador
swish	hacer buches
swollen	hinchado(a)
symptom	el síntoma
syringe	la jeringa
syrup	el jarabe
tablespoon	la cuchara
tablespoonful	la cucharada
tablet	la tableta
to take	tomar
to take, to carry	llevar
to take away, to take out	retirar
to take out	sacar
to take time	tardar
talc, powder (skin)	el talco
to talk	hablar
tampon	el tampón
taste buds	las papilas gustativas
tearduct	el lagrimal
tearful, weeping	lloroso(a)
teaspoon	la cucharita
teaspoonful	la cucharadita
temperature	la temperatura
temples	las sienes
temporarily	temporalmente
tense	tenso(a)
tension	la tensión
testicle	el testículo
tetanus	el tétanos
there is, there are (impersonal)	hay
thermometer	el termómetro
thick	espeso(a), viscoso(a)
thick, solid	sólido(a), duro(a)
thigh	el muslo
thin	delgado(a)
thin, lazy	flojo(a)
thing	la cosa
to think	pensar
thirst	la sed
thoroughly	a fondo
throat	la garganta

Thursday	el jueves
thyroid	la tiroides
tight-fitting	apretado(a)
tight squeeze	el apretón
to tilt, to lean	inclinar(se)
time	el tiempo
to tingle (like ants)	hormiguear
tingling (like ants)	el hormigueo
tinnitus (ringing)	el tinnitus
toe	el dedo del pie
toenails	las uñas de los pies
toilet paper	el papel higiénico, el papel sanitario
tolerable	tolerable
tongue	la lengua
tonsils	las anginas
too much	demasiado(a)
too, also	también
tooth	el diente
top of the foot	el empeine del pie
topical	tópico(a)
to touch	tocar
tourist-like	turístico(a)
toward	hacia
toxicity	la toxicidad
trachea	la tráquea
tragus, "earflap"	la lengüeta de la oreja, el trago
transparent	transparente
trash	la basura
trashcan	el cesto de la basura
to travel	viajar
treatment	el tratamiento
tricuspid	tricúspide
troche	el trocisco
to try, to treat (illness)	tratar
tube	el tubo
tuberculosis	la tuberculosis
Tuesday	el martes
tympannic membrane	el tímpano
type	el tipo
ulcer	la úlcera
uncomfortable	incómodo(a)
under	(a)bajo, (de)bajo
underweight	bajo de peso
unit(s)	la(s) unidad(es)
up, above	arriba
urethra	la uretra
to urinate	orinar
urine	la pipí (euphemism)
urticaria	la urticaria
to use	usar
usual diet	la alimentación
usually	usualmente, de costumbre
uterus	el útero, la matriz
to utilize	utilizar
uvula	la campanilla
to vacuum	aspirar, la úvula

vagina	la vagina	to walk	caminar	whitish	blancuzco(a)
vaginal discharge	el flujo vaginal	wall	la pared	whole-grain bread	el pan integral
vaginal suppository	el óvulo vaginal	to want	querer	window	la ventana
valve	la válvula	warning	la advertencia	winter	el invierno
Vaseline®,	la vaselina	wart	el mezquino	with	con
petroleum jelly		to wash	lavar(se)	withdrawal	el síndrome de
vegetable	la verdura, el	to watch	observar		abstinencia
	vegetal	water fountain	el bebedero	without	sin
vein	la vena	watery	aguado(a)	without fat	desgrasado(a)
ventricle	el ventrículo	weakness	la debilidad	word	la palabra
vertigo	el vértigo	Wednesday	el miércoles	to worry	preocupar(se)
very	muy	week	la semana	worse	peor
very much	muchísimo(a)	weekend(s)	el fín de semana	to worsen	empeorar
vial	el frasco ámpula		(los fines de	wound	la herida
vial, small bottle	el frasco		semana)	wrapper	la envoltura
viral	viral (de virus)	to weigh	pesar	wrist	la muñeca
to vomit	vomitar	weight	el peso	wrong, mistaken	equivocado(a)
vomit	el vómito	wet	mojado(a)	year	el año
vulva	la vulva	wheezing	el silbido	yellow	amarillo(a)
waist	la cintura	while	mientras	yellowish	amarillento(a)
to wait	esperar	white	blanco(a)	your own	propio(a)
to wake up	despertar(se)	whitehead	el punto blanco	zone	la zona